The Home Apothecary

© 2013 by Quarry Books
Text © 2013 Stacey Dugliss-Wesselman
Photography © 2013 Chris Pinkus Wesselman

First published in the United States of America in 2013 by
Quarry Books, a member of
Quarto Publishing Group USA Inc
100 Cummings Center
Suite 406-L
Beverly, Massachusetts 01915-6101
Telephone: (978) 282-9590
Fax: (978) 283-2742
www.quarrybooks.com

10 9 8 7 6 5 4

ISBN: 978-1-59253-819-5

Digital edition published in 2013
eISBN: 978-1-61058-769-3

Library of Congress Cataloging-in-Publication Data is available

Page Design: Rita Sowins / Sowins Design

Printed in China

The Home Apothecary

Cold Spring Apothecary's Cookbook of
Hand-Crafted Remedies & Recipes
for the Hair, Skin, Body, and Home

★ Stacey Dugliss-Wesselman ★

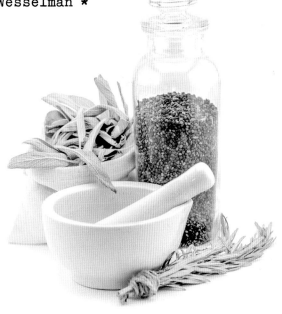

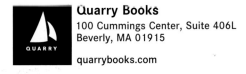

Quarry Books
100 Cummings Center, Suite 406L
Beverly, MA 01915

quarrybooks.com

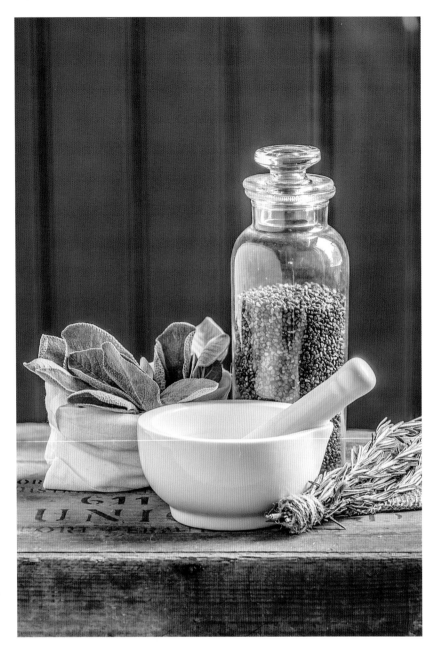

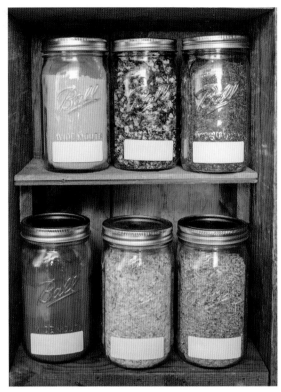

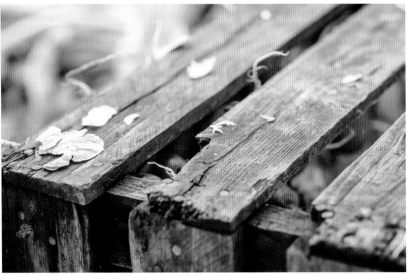

CONTENTS

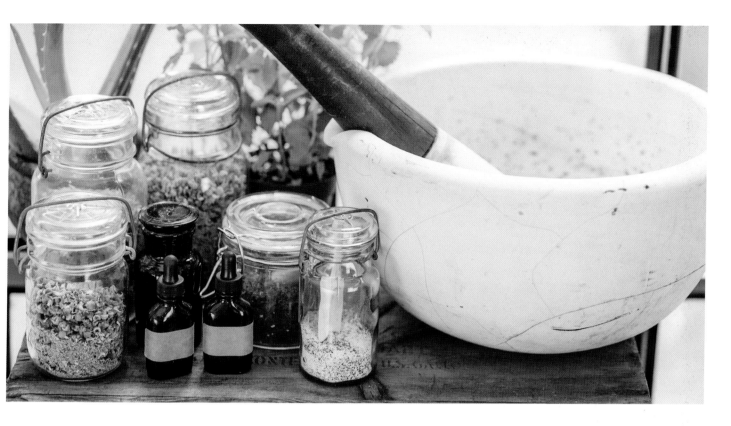

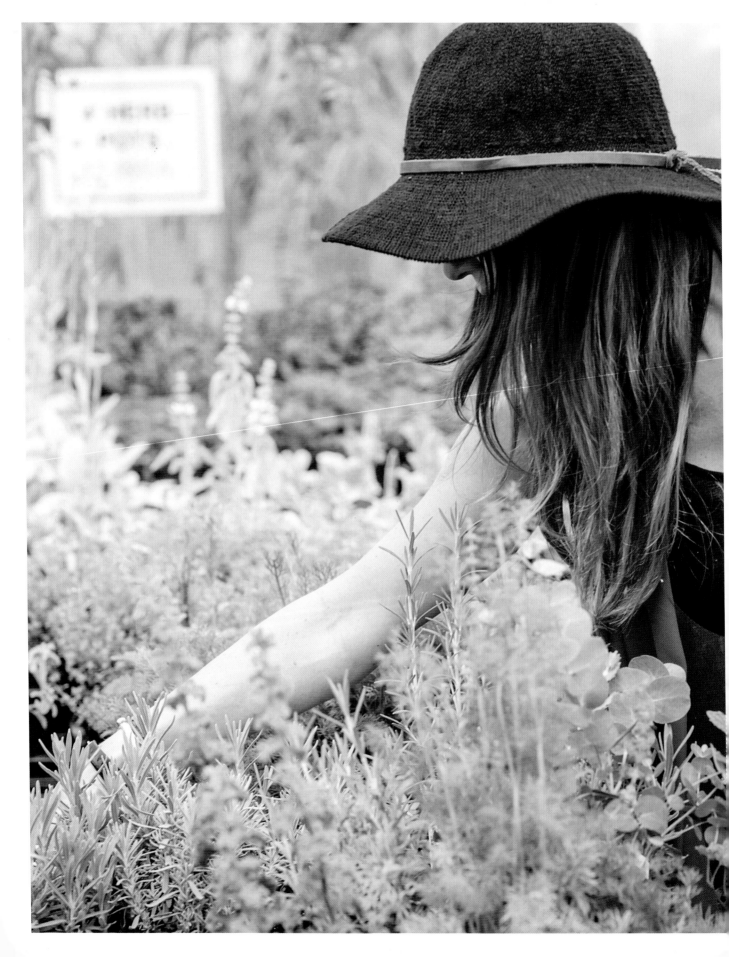

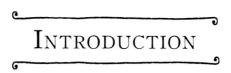

INTRODUCTION

TODAY, NATURALS PLAY A VERY IMPORTANT ROLE IN MY LIFE, BUT THIS WASN'T ALWAYS THE CASE. Since as far back as I can remember, the natural world has always amazed me. I'd spend hours in the wilderness foraging for plants, herbs, and just about anything that looked interesting, and then equally as many hours looking through books to figure out what I had found. Back then I never knew I could use these found treasures to make cosmetics or to heal ailments. It wasn't until my teenage years, when the closest store wasn't so close at all, that I started mixing things in the kitchen to create last-minute beauty fixes. Although not all my kitchen chemistry went as planned, I learned that creating your own cosmetics was not only thrifty but also rewarding. The power to create something natural with your hands to heal yourself was nothing short of magic to me.

While my teenaged years allowed for experimentation with naturals, my adult life proved far too busy for kitchen healing and cosmetics. It was too easy to run to the store and grab a lotion from a shelf filled with colorful bottles promising to make me beautiful.

My true love of naturals came out of necessity. While living in New York City, my skin went from flawless to far from it. I started getting adult acne, and I tried product after product to no avail. Frustrated and embarrassed, I started reading all I could about skin care. It was through this quest for knowledge that I found my return to kitchen cosmetics. The healing power of herbs fascinated me, and again I started experimenting with essential oils in my existing over-the-counter products. It wasn't until I started making my cosmetics completely from scratch that I saw a complete change in my skin. What was in the over-the-counter products that I was using, and how were they affecting my skin? My research only made me regret the years I'd spent slathering harmful chemicals all over my skin and hair. It was around this same time that I began my career as a hairstylist and discovered that most of my clientele had similar complaints and concerns about their daily skin care and hair care regimens. I started mixing my concoctions for my clients, and after rave reviews, I quit my job, moved to the Hudson Valley, and locked myself in a room for two years, learning and mixing all I could.

From this, Cold Spring Apothecary was born. What began with shampoo turned into a complete hair care line, and it has continued to expand. My vision was to create a natural healthful base with additional active naturals to create treatments for various ailments. I started off with what I knew best, essential oils, but have since expanded to other active naturals and treatments. With so many naturals on the market and with ingredients constantly evolving, there is always more to learn and improve.

The focus of this book is much the same. I've laid the groundwork for your experiments with naturals. You'll soon find that not every recipe will work out for you the first time, but over time you will easily master kitchen cosmetics, begin to create your own recipes, and find naturals that work for you. All the recipes are starting points and can be altered to your needs. I encourage you to research as much information as you can; there are so many great books and resources out there about naturals. You'll come across tons of similar base recipes and you, too, will be able to make them your own.

PART I

Become a Home Apothecary

*

"And thou shalt make it a perfume,
a confection after the art of the Apothecary,
tempered together, pure and holy."

— *Exodus 30:35*

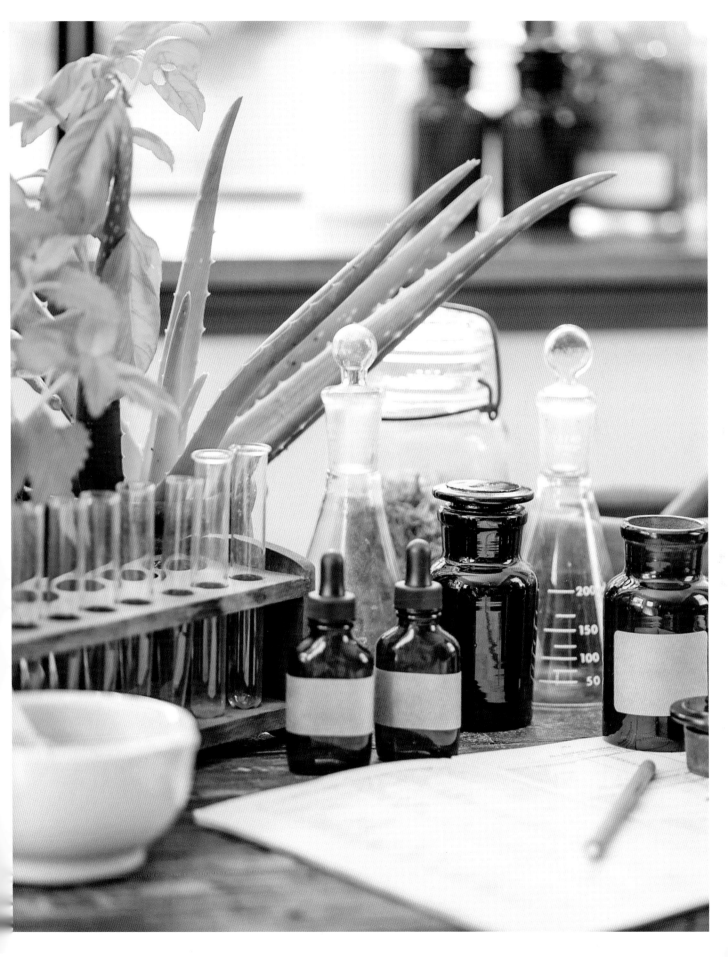

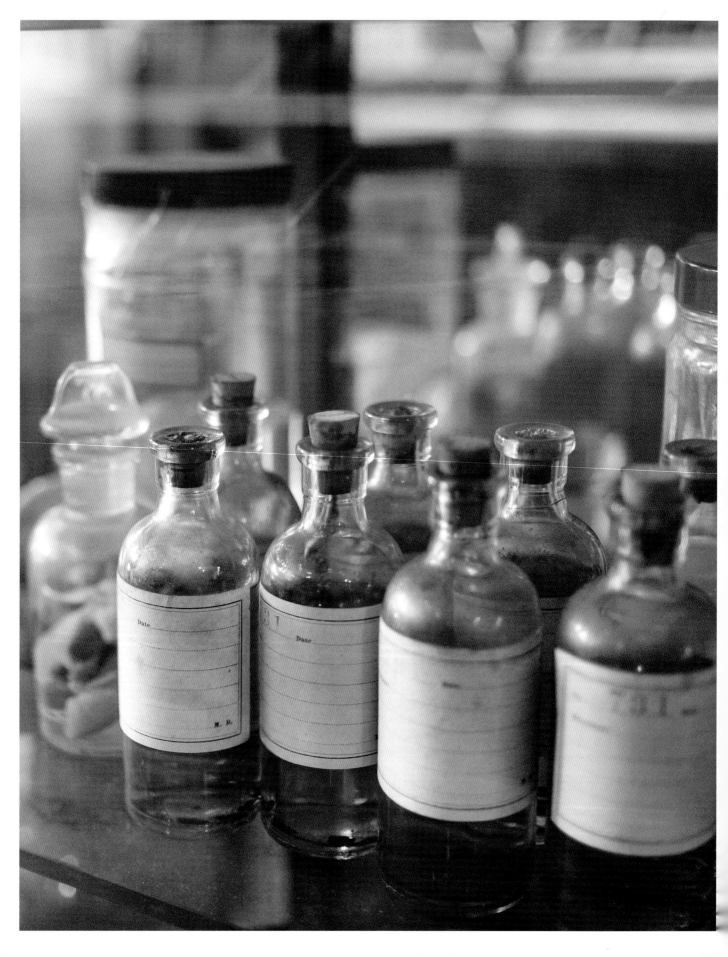

CHAPTER 1

Meet the Apothecaries

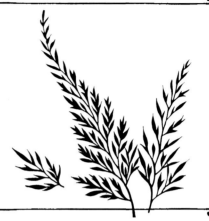

OFTEN CONFUSED WITH A PLACE, AN APOTHECARY IS A SKILLED CRAFTSPERSON WHO PREPARES COMPOUNDS FOR A MEDICINAL OBJECTIVE. THE CRAFT OF USING HERBS TO ENHANCE OUR HEALTH AND BEAUTY HAS BEEN AROUND FOR DECADES. IN A MODERN WORLD OF TRICKY MARKETING AND CHEMICAL-LADEN PRODUCTS, WE ARE SLOWLY FINDING OUR WAY BACK TO NATURE AND ALL THAT IT HAS TO OFFER.

A BRIEF HISTORY OF THE APOTHECARY'S CRAFT

An apothecary is a skilled craftsperson who compounds herbal and mineral mixtures to treat ailments. Our use of herbs (also known as herbalism), oils, minerals, and later even animal and human ingredients, can be traced to as early as 2250 BCE; tablets with recorded recipes of herbs for the treatment of ailments have been dated back that far. This act of using nature to cure our ills most likely began out of necessity and by some luck. To cover a painful burn, for instance, we used a leaf which then produced a numbing effect. Or perhaps we watched other animals around us consume certain plants after appearing sick, and we then found that eating those plants eased an upset stomach. Over time, and most likely by trial and error, we learned that plants could affect our bodies with hallucinogenic, analgesic, antibacterial, and laxative effects.

As our knowledge of nature's ability to heal advanced, so did the art of the apothecary. Over time and from culture to culture, natural medicinal recipes were created and shared. These recipes were then passed on and added to in each following generation. Eventually, herbs and minerals were used to create topical and internal concoctions, tinctures, medicinal wines, poultices, lotions, and salves. With the addition of mysticism and astrology to the recipes, shamans and village healers became known for using nature's bounty for their treatments. Similarly, herbalists mixed the use of herbs with astrology.

Herbalists became gardeners—they focused not only on a plant's usage but also on the effect of the soil, the lunar cycle, and the rain on the plant's medicinal strength.

Traditionally, women prepared the compounds. It was women who used herbalism most often as a way of life, providing for both family and village. However, it was men who carried on these medicinal traditions and recipes over time; therefore, men were most often credited with their results.

The art of the apothecary advanced with the limited scientific knowledge of the time, and apothecaries became highly regarded figures, much like today's physicians, while using their herbal therapeutics to treat the ill. They added chemical procedures learned from alchemists to their herbal compounds. Eventually opening shops much like general stores, they sold perfumes and tobacco, and even on occasion diagnosed diseases. Apothecaries were categorized as or lumped in with grocers and spicers.

With advancements in the field of medical science, physicians sought to do away with apothecaries. Like the modern-day pharmacist, the apothecary prepared the compounds that the practitioner prescribed. This is where the confusion over the apothecary as a place—as a pharmacy—comes from. Then came pharmaceutical companies, and with them the demise of what once was the apothecary craft.

The apothecaries' combined studies in herbalism and alchemy can very easily be thought of as laying the groundwork for the modern sciences of chemistry and pharmacology. Their advanced studies in botany allow herbalists and modern-day apothecaries to succeed today with the ever-growing desire for natural alternatives. And they have influenced modern medical science as well: According to the World Health Organization, nearly 25 percent of modern drugs' curative effects are derived from plant extracts. But it wasn't until 2004 that the National Center for Complementary and Alternative Medicine started to fund clinical trials to evaluate the effectiveness of herbal medicine.

The apothecaries were artists, and unlike the pharmacies of today that are so far removed from the creation of their dispensed remedies, they had a dedication and passion for nature's cures.

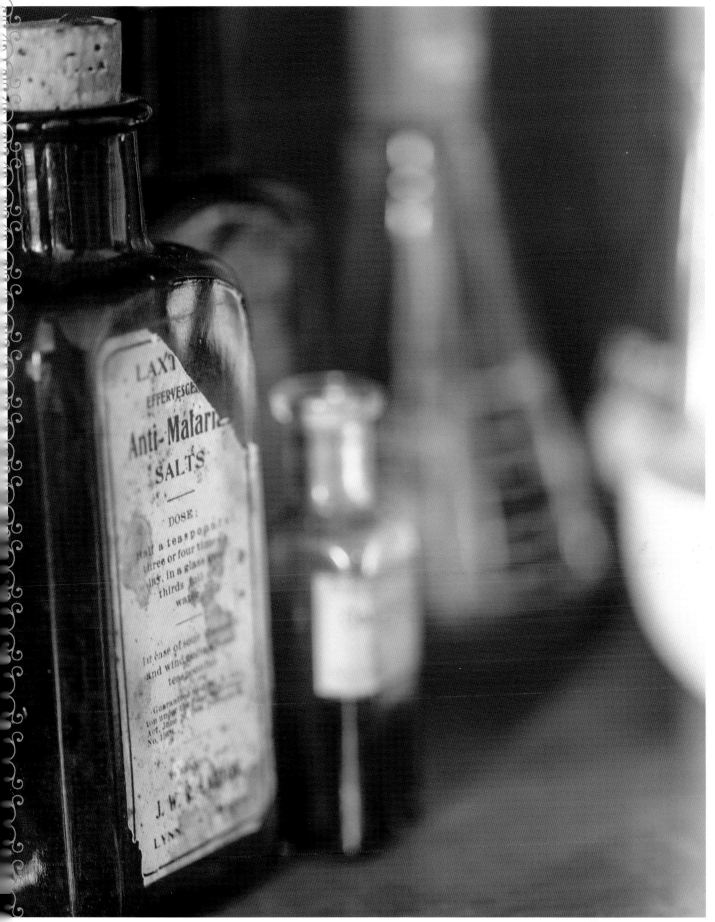

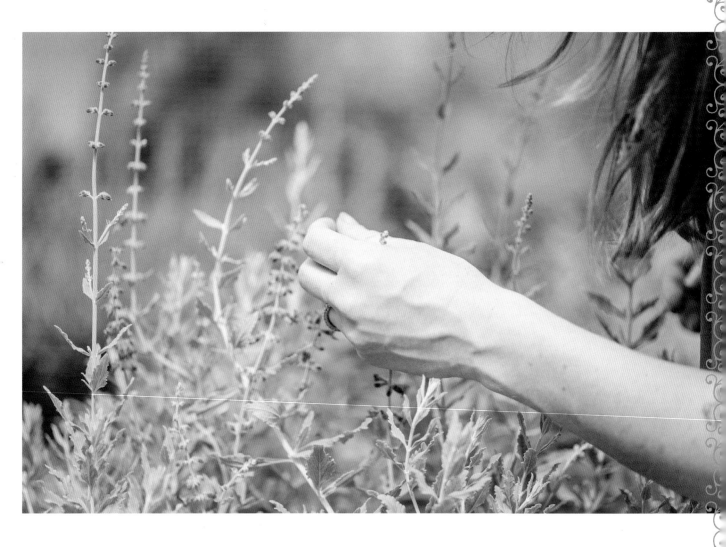

The Importance of Naturals

Beauty and health are an age-old quest. Unfortunately, in modern times our beauty solutions have not exactly been the healthiest for us.

In our vanity we have also become lazy, opting for easier, quicker solutions like diet pills, cosmetics, and even surgical forms of beauty preparations and treatments.

Long before laboratory research and technology, botany and medicine went hand in hand. The plant life around us has long been used for both medicinal and vanity purposes to better our lives. With the advancement of modern science, "natural medicine" has often been disregarded, and it has gained negative connotations. Sadly, modern medicines and beauty preparations are often focused on only one ailment or remedy, while a single herb can treat a variety of things. Nature's herbs and oils treat us internally and externally.

Although we tend to be slightly more mindful about what we put in our bodies, we don't often think about what we put *on* them. But what we put on our skin and hair goes into our bodies. Researchers say that the body absorbs up to 60 percent of what we put on our skin—our biggest organ. With new products coming onto the market every day that claim to penetrate the skin faster, we should be aware of the hazards that may be penetrating it with them.

Mainstream cosmetic products often contain toxic ingredients such as carcinogens, endocrine disrupters, and allergens. A carcinogen is a substance that causes cancer. An endocrine disrupter mimics or interferes with the body's hormones and can cause reproductive or neurological damage.

The main problem is that we use so many products with so many ingredients. The average American woman uses twelve products daily (men use six), with upward of 168 ingredients (85 for men) total. Further, we use them for long periods of time; although a deodorant containing carcinogenic ingredients may not harm you with one use, you mostly likely won't use deodorant only once in your life.

We often put far too much faith in regulatory agencies to make sure our products are safe. For instance, the U.S. Food and Drug Administration (FDA) leaves it up to the cosmetic industry to regulate itself. In other words, if it makes money and is cheap to produce, why change it regardless of its effects? At a 1997 hearing on the FDA reform bill, the late senator Edward Kennedy warned that the "cosmetic industry has borrowed a page from the playbook of the tobacco industry by putting profits ahead of public health." What the FDA terms "generally recognized as safe" doesn't necessarily mean safe as in lab-tested, but safe as in consumer-tested—meaning already commonly used in consumer products.

There are also very limited restrictions on labeling and claims. Companies are allowed to leave certain ingredients or "trade secrets" off of packaging. Just because it's not on the label doesn't mean it's not in the product. Also, with increased awareness of our desire for healthier, natural products, big industry has created a bit of "natural" product confusion, manipulating us into purchasing their so-called natural products by using gimmicks and catchphrases. A product can contain less than 1 percent natural ingredients—say, a few drops of lavender oil—and still market itself as "natural" regardless of what else is in it.

The bottom line is, education is key. Read the label and know what harmful ingredients to be mindful of. Don't assume that regulatory agencies will be responsible and warn us. Just because it's an over-the-counter product or marketed as making us more youthful and healthful doesn't mean it's safe or that it has been tested for its long-term safety effects.

On the next page are a few of the commonly used harmful ingredients found in cosmetic products today. There are plenty of websites that offer more comprehensive listings, and I strongly urge you to research any ingredients you run across. But remember, just because a product has a long name (often its required Latin name) doesn't mean it's harmful. If you have a question, just research it—even things that are naturally derived may not be safe alternatives to what's in use today. Be educated!

Harmful Ingredient	Effects
Parabens are a class of chemicals widely used as preservatives in the cosmetic industry; they include methyl, propyl, butyl, and ethyl.	Endocrine disruptors that have been linked to cancer; environmental contaminants.
Sodium laureth sulfate and **sodium lauryl sulfate**, which are used as surfactants, or "lather agents," in most shampoos, are found in most cosmetic products on the market today because they are an inexpensive ingredient and make mass production cheaper. Consumers have become accustomed to "suds" in their cleansers.	Known skin and eye irritants; environmental contaminants. Not only are they harmful, but they are also extremely drying to the hair and skin.
Phthalates (**DBP, DEP, DEHP, and DMP**) are most often used to create fragrances in cosmetic products.	Endocrine disruptors.
Boric acid is considered an antiseptic and a fungicide. Used in many cosmetic and medicinal products.	Reproductive toxin; endocrine disruptor.
Bronopol is used as a preservative in a wide variety of cosmetics and toiletries.	Lung and skin toxin; endocrine disruptor; carcinogen.
Butylated hydroxyanisole (**BHA**) and **butylated hydroxytoluene** (**BHT**) are preservatives and antioxidants used in cosmetics and foods.	Allergens; endocrine disrupters; possible carcinogens.
Coal tar is used to make many dyes, so be aware of products with dyes in them.	Carcinogen; skin irritant.
Formaldehyde has many uses but is most often used in cosmetics as a disinfectant and preservative. Also be aware of products containing **1,4-dioxane**, because this can release formaldehyde in certain chemical processes.	Carcinogen; skin, eye, and lung irritant; organ irritant.
Imidazolidinyl urea (**uric acid**) is a common preservative in cosmetics.	Skin and eye irritate; endocrine disruptor.
Polyethylene glycol (**PEG**) is a binder and plasticizing ingredient used in a wide variety of cosmetics.	Endocrine disrupter.
Talc is used in baby and body powders (talcum powder) as an astringent.	Skin and lung irritant; carcinogen.
Thioglycolic acid is used in perms, straighteners, and depilatories.	Skin and lung irritant.

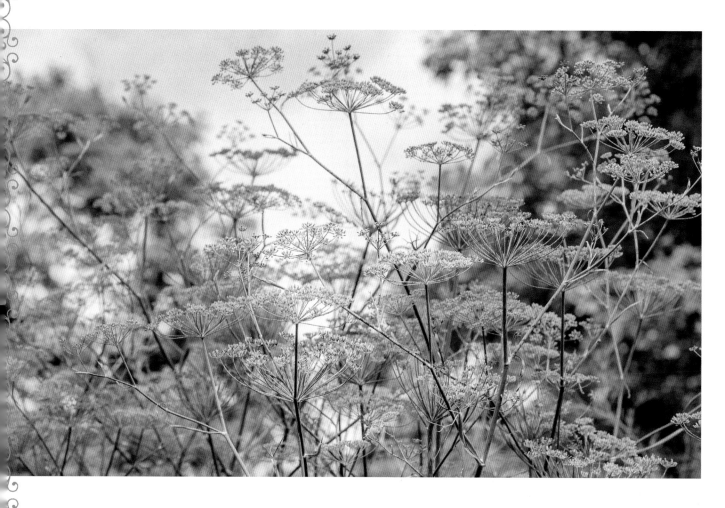

Taking care of your body and home by using naturals will not only cut down on the number of chemicals you put into your body but can also save you money.

By making your own products, you can control the ingredients used, scent to your preferences, and customize to your skin's needs. Nature has given us all we need for both inner and outer health; we just need to explore it. For example, creating a lotion with fennel will not only treat bruises, combat oily skin, and aid in the prevention of wrinkles, but also its aromatherapy properties are said to elicit courage and strengthen resolve. It also has numerous internal medicinal properties. It's great when used as an after-dinner gentle cleansing tea, helps promote fullness, and acts as a diuretic.

This book will teach you how herbalists and apothecaries use nature to combine both health and beauty—and how you can, too.

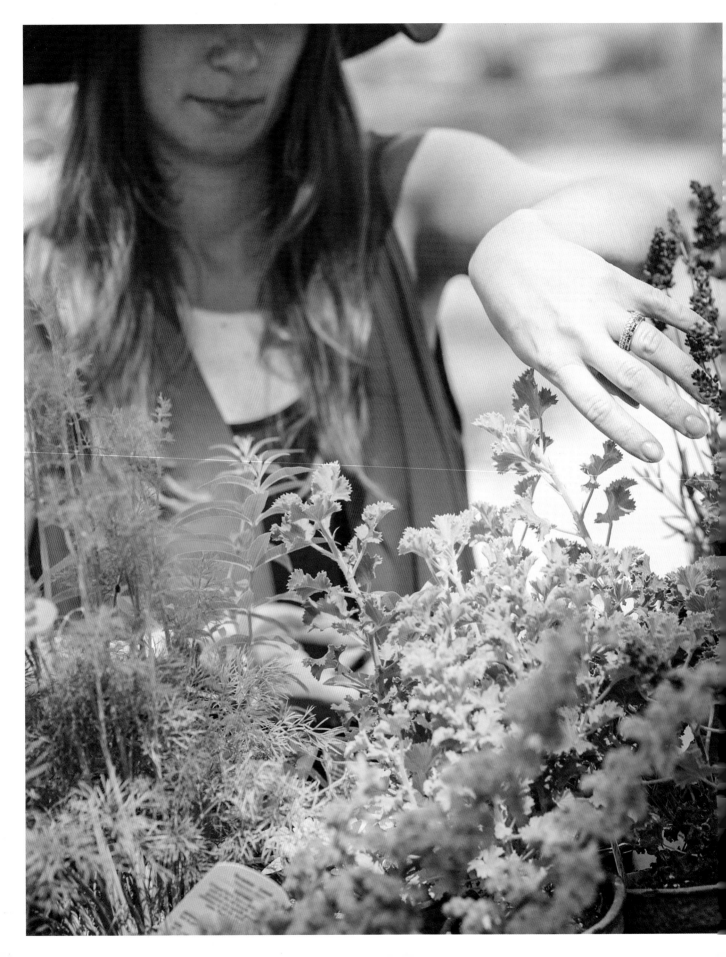

CHAPTER 2

Set Up an Apothecary Pantry

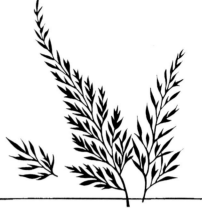

Whether you plan on foraging for your herbs, growing them in your garden, or purchasing them from an organic vendor, once you've selected all your natural ingredients and gathered your supplies, you're ready to become an apothecary. This chapter will help you navigate your way through selecting the herbs and other active natural ingredients you'll need to create your kitchen concoctions.

Essential Oils

Essential oils have many uses and are found in cosmetics, foods, medicines, and aromatherapy. They can help diminish the signs of aging, heal a scar, or disinfect your kitchen counter. And they are quite valuable in skin and hair care preparations because of their ability to penetrate the skin with their many benefits.

Essential oils are extractions made from flowers, grasses, fruits, leaves, roots, and trees. There are many different extraction methods, including steam distillation, solvent extraction, expression, effleurage, and maceration. The method most often depends on the species. Contrary to their name, essential oils are not oils at all, because they don't contain essential fatty acids. Therefore, they shouldn't leave behind a greasy feel and when dripped on paper shouldn't leave an oil spot.

Essentials oils are very precious because it can sometimes take a large quantity of a particular species to produce only a few drops of the oil. For that reason, you should be aware when purchasing them. A good sign of a quality oil company is different prices for different oils; if rose otto is the same price as lavender, that's a sign that something is wrong. Be sure to purchase from a reputable vendor, and make sure your purchases are 100 percent essential oil and not some type of synthetic or perfumery copy. Especially when you are purchasing an essential oil for therapeutic use, a mixture of essentials to create the scent of another essential oil will not have the therapeutic effect of that oil. Try to purchase organic when it's available to you.

You should purchase and store your oils in dark amber vials in a cool area away from direct sunlight. Unless you plan on using large amounts of oils or are making cosmetics, you should try to purchase oils in smaller quantities to ensure freshness over time.

While the many uses of essential oils may be impressive, it can also be overwhelming. It's best to start off with a few you are comfortable with and build from there. There are many types of essential oils, and you should research the uses and precautions for each one prior to using it. Some oils can't be applied to the skin neat and should always be mixed with carrier oil, some shouldn't be used by babies and children or during pregnancy, and some make you more sensitive to sunlight. It is advised and always best to use only pure essential oils externally unless otherwise instructed by a doctor or health care professional.

Below are some of my favorites, including ones that I use throughout the recipes in this book. But any of the recipes can be altered to suit your needs or scent preferences as you begin to expand your essential oil knowledge.

⇢ QUICK FIRST-AID OILS ⇠

* **Abrasions:** Lavender, tea tree, neroli, frankincense, myrrh.

* **Black eyes:** Chamomile, lavender, rose. Dilute a few drops of any of these with some witch hazel and apply to area (avoid getting into eyes).

* **Blisters:** Lavender, chamomile, lemon, tea tree.

* **Bruises:** Geranium, lavender, parsley, rosemary. Make a compress using gauze and dilute a few drops of any of these in witch hazel.

* **Cold sores:** Geranium, lemon, tea tree, thyme. Dilute a few drops of one or a combination in grapeseed oil.

* **Headaches:** Chamomile, coriander, lavender, peppermint, rosemary. Massage the hairline with a few drops of one or a combination diluted in jojoba oil.

* **Insect bites:** Apply a drop of lavender to the affected area.

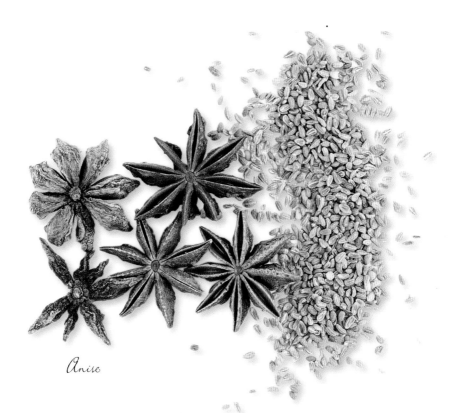

Anise

Angelica *(Angelica archangelica)*: Sweet, herbal, peppery scent. Grounding and calming; relieves anxiety. Helps fight infections, stimulating the immune system and acting as an expectorant to remove toxins from the body.

* *

Anise *(Pimpinella anisum)*: Aids in digestion. Energizes the mind. Can be used to treat acne, muscle aches, cramps, and colds. Anise should never be applied to the skin neat without a carrier oil.

* *

Basil, sweet *(Ocimum basilicum)*: Floral aroma with an herbal, licorice sweetness. Immune-system stimulating, this oil has both anti-inflammatory and antibacterial properties. Great when used in insect repellents or even to treat bites. Basil is an antidepressant and helps promote concentration.

* *

Bay laurel *(Laurus nobilis)*: Earthy tone. Eases aches and pains. Great for use in hair tonics for dandruff or oily hair.

Bergamot *(Styrax benzoin)*, **bergaptene-free:** Fresh, citrusy, and uplifting aroma. Great for oily or acne-prone skin; has antiseptic properties. Acts as an antidepressant, lifting the spirits. Be advised that this oil reacts to sunlight.

* *

Black willow bark *(Salix nigra)*: This herb has aspirin-like chemicals, making it good for treating headaches and fevers. Its antimicrobial properties help treat acne-prone skin.

* *

Calendula *(Calendula officinalis)*: A great medicinal oil; has long history in the both skin care recipes and wound care ointments. Rich in antioxidants; great for treating dry and damaged skin, skin inflammations, burns, rashes, and other skin disorders.

* *

Camphor *(Cinnamomum camphora)*: A clean, strong, medicinal aroma. Analgesic and antiseptic; great for sore muscles or inflammation when used in salves for overworked muscles and joints. This oil is strong, and only a small amount is needed to feel the effects.

* *

Carrot seed *(Daucus carota)*: Don't be fooled by its name—this oil doesn't smell like carrots, but has a sweet vegetable scent. High levels of vitamins A, C, and B_1 make this a favorite for serums and lotions for mature skin, fighting the signs of aging. It helps with many skin disorders, such as eczema and psoriasis, and helps smooth scars. Its effects aren't just on the skin; it's great in hair tonics to help thicken and add shine.

* *

Cedarwood, Atlas *(Cedrus atlantica)*: Fresh, woodsy smell. Has many uses for hair, skin, and aromatherapy. Great for skin irritations like eczema, psoriasis, and acne. Helps clear the respiratory system and eases anxiety. Works great in insect repellents.

* *

Chamomile *(Matricaria recutita)*: Distinct herbal scent. There are several different types of chamomile essential oil, and it's a good one to always have on hand. Known for its calming and soothing effects, but not so commonly known as an antibacterial and a disinfectant; gentle enough for sensitive skin types and children (Roman chamomile [*Anthemis nobilis*] is best). Mix a little with lavender oil and it's great to treat an itchy bug bite. It works wonders on dry itchy skin, or for those with eczema or psoriasis. You don't need a lot to feel its effects.

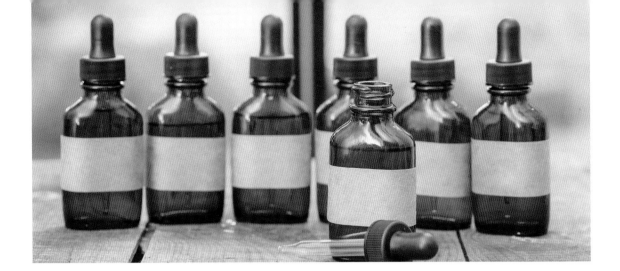

Cinnamon (*Cinnamomum zeylanicum*) (leaf is milder; bark is stronger): Strong, sharp smell. Useful in the treatment of insect bite irritation as well as in insect sprays to kill lice. Antibacterial and antifungal. Stimulates circulation and lowers stress in aromatherapy blends. Use caution when using cinnamon leaf or bark in skin applications, because it can be irritating to the skin. Avoid if you are prone to headaches.

* *

Clary sage (*Salvia sclarea*): Spicy, earthy, herbal, bittersweet scent. Known for its aromatherapy powers and to lift the spirits. Great for women to ease premenstrual mood swings, and men will enjoy its stress-relieving aroma. Add a few drops to your favorite shampoo or conditioner for an uplifting and centering morning shower. Works wonders when added to a winter salve to remedy asthma or coughing. A word of caution when using clary sage: its sedative effects are strong, and overuse can even cause a somewhat intoxicated state. Also, its shouldn't be used when pregnant or breastfeeding.

* *

Clove (*Eugenia caryophyllata*): Strong, spicy aroma. Uplifting; helps improve memory function; eases bronchial irritations. Works well for toothaches.

* *

Cypress (*Cupressus sempervirens*): Fresh pine-like scent. Great for soothing varicose veins, eczema, and oily skin. It is also a great deodorant and an antiseptic. Helps clear the mind.

* *

Dill (*Anethum sowa*): Grassy scent. Helpful in the treatment of digestive issues such as flatulence, constipation, and even hiccups. Calms the mind, easing headaches and tension.

* *

Elemi (*Canarium luzonicum*): Spicy, citrusy aroma. Useful in treatment of bronchial irritations. Regulates perspiration and balances sebum. Can also be used on cuts, wounds, and skin infections. Its aroma helps relax the nerves and ease stress. Great as a room refresher.

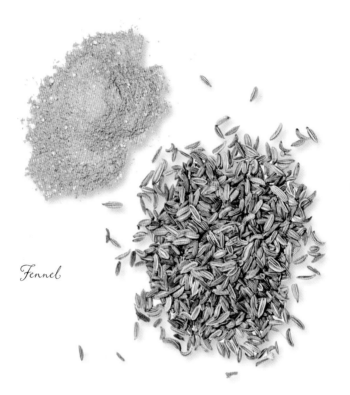

Fennel

Eucalyptus *(Eucalyptus globulus)*: Cool, menthol scent. There are several types of eucalyptus. Has antiseptic, antifungal, expectorant, and deodorizing properties. Great to use as a bug repellent and even in bite treatment recipes. Works well on aches and pains.

* *

Fennel *(Foeniculum vulgare)*: Licorice-like scent. Aids in digestion and helps increase circulation. Useful in healing bruises, correcting oily skin, and fighting wrinkles.

* *

Frankincense *(Boswellia carteri)*: An uplifting, spicy, woodsy scent. Great for dry, mature skin as well as oily blemish-prone skin types. Adding this oil to your lotions helps with scars and stretch marks. Its relaxing aroma helps ease anxiety.

* *

Ginger *(Zingiber officinale)*: Warm, spicy aroma. As an antibacterial and analgesic, ginger works on achy muscles, arthritis, poor circulation, and nausea. Its aroma is uplifting and energizing.

* *

Grapefruit *(Citrus paradisi)*: Citrus fragrance. Great for lifting the spirits. Its powers don't stop at aromatherapy: grapefruit also helps rid the body of toxins and helps eliminate water weight and cellulite.

Helichrysum (*Helichrysum angustifolium*): Herbal, fruity smell. Anti-inflammatory, astringent, analgesic, and an expectorant. Helpful for circulatory disorders, improving blood flow. Beneficial effect on colds, flu, bronchitis, coughs, and asthma. Has superb regenerating qualities and can assist in the healing of scars, acne, and stretch marks.

* *

Jasmine (*Jasminum officinale*): Sweet, floral, and rich aroma. Helps calm and nourish dry skin and fights signs of aging. Aroma is relaxing and calming to the nerves.

* *

Juniper (*Juniperus communis*): Woodsy, green scent. Antiseptic, astringent, diuretic, and detoxifying agent. Great for cellulite treatments, swelling, and eliminating toxins from the body. Excellent for skin care and helps unblock the pores, treating acne, eczema, and psoriasis.

* *

Lavender (*Lavandula officinalis*): Refreshing floral scent. This very versatile oil is used to treat a variety of conditions, from skin irritations, burns, bug bites, and acne to relieving stress, anxiety, depression, and insomnia.

* *

Lemon (*Citrus limonum*): Fresh, citrusy scent. Disinfecting; used in cleansers and to eliminate odors. Refreshing aroma helps ease depression, stress, and anxiety.

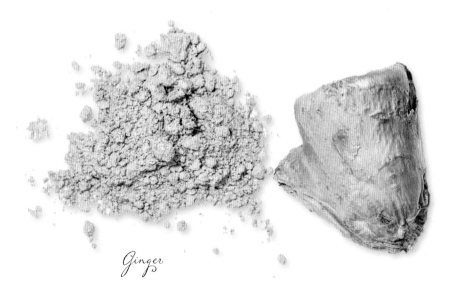

Ginger

Lemongrass *(Cymbopogon flexuosus)*: Green citrus scent. Lemongrass helps oily skin, reducing pore size. It also acts as a natural insect repellent.

* *

Lime *(Citrus aurantifolia)*: Fruity, citrusy aroma. Uplifting and refreshing, lime revitalizes the mind. Great for oily skin types. Also works as a disinfectant.

* *

Mandarin *(Citrus reticulata)*: Sweet citrus scent. A great antiseptic; works well on acne-prone and sensitive skin.

* *

Myrrh *(Commiphora myrrha)*: Warm, sweet, musty, resin scent. Has anti-inflammatory, antiseptic, and disinfectant properties. Helps clear bronchial irritation and congestion. It's also used to treat mouth and gum disorders. In skin care recipes, myrrh helps chapped and cracked skin, eczema, and skin sores.

* *

Neroli *(Citrus aurantium)*: Floral, citrusy scent. Great for all skin types; can be used to treat acne, regenerate skin cells, prevent scar tissue, and fight stretch marks.

* *

Niaouli *(Melaleuca quinquenervia)*: Pungent, earthy aroma. Most often used medicinally to treat colds and respiratory infections. Has analgesic, antiseptic, and expectorant properties. Works well on oily skin prone to acne. Helps with circulation and sore muscles.

* *

Palmarosa *(Cymbopogon martini)*: Sweet, floral, tea-like aroma. Has antibacterial, antifungal, and antiseptic properties. On the skin, it's great for acne, eczema, scar tissue, and wrinkles. Palmarosa also works well as an insect repellent. Its aroma is quite often used in perfumes but acts as a stimulant.

* *

Patchouli *(Pogostemon patchouli)*: Musky, woodsy, pungent aroma. This oil is used as an anti-inflammatory, an antiseptic, and a deodorant. Patchouli works great on all skin types, soothing dry skin and balancing oils. It's also a great to use in hair care recipes for cleansing dry scalp and dandruff. Its aroma is believed to be an antidepressant, and both a stimulant and a sedative.

* *

Peppermint *(Mentha piperita)*: Strong, clean, menthol scent. One of the more commonly known and used oils. When used internally, it can calm an upset stomach, relieve flatulence, and ease motion sickness. Due to its antiseptic properties, it is great for use in toothpastes and mouthwashes. Topically, it nourishes dull skin and improves oily skin. When used in hair care recipes, it helps with dandruff and kills lice. Peppermint oil is also used as a headache cure, to treat respiratory issues, and to ease stress.

* *

Peru balsam *(Myroxylon pereirae)*: Dark brown oil with a sweet, earthy smell. Lovely in fragrance blends, especially more masculine blends. Works great on those with irritated skin issues such as eczema, dermatitis, and rashes.

* *

Petitgrain *(Citrus aurantium)*: Woodsy, citrusy scent with a hint of floral. A great oil for oily, acne-prone skin but gentle enough for all skin types to help regulate and tone the skin. Lovely in lotions and body oils. Its uplifting aroma clears confusion and relaxes and calms the nerves.

* *

Pine *(Pinus sylvestris)*: Clean, woodsy aroma. Naturally deodorizing and a disinfectant, pine oil can be used in skin care, aromatherapy, and to make household cleaning products.

* *

Ravensara *(Ravensara aromatica)*: Slightly spicy, woodsy aroma. Great for bronchial irritation and congestion. Helps fight fever and flu as well as muscular aches and pains.

* *

Rose *(Rosa damascena)*: Sweet floral aroma. A favorite for perfumery, rose is an antidepressant, uplifting and stimulating the spirits. It has been used for centuries in skin care preparations for its antiaging, skin-healing properties. You can use either rose otto or rose absolute. Rose otto is usually more expensive because it is steam distilled and most often preferred by aromatherapists or for use in cosmetic applications. Rose absolute is solvent extracted and is most often preferred by perfumers.

* *

Rose geranium *(Pelargonium graveolens)*: Sweet and rosy smell. One of my favorite oils for skin care preparations, it works great on all skin types and gives skin radiance, helps regulate oily skin, fight cellulite, and relieve pain.

* *

Rosemary *(Rosmarinus officinalis)*: Herbal, fresh scent. This oil is an antiseptic, astringent, and cerebral stimulant. Helps with indigestion, bad breath, respiratory problems, and pain relief. An amazing oil for the hair, rosemary helps stimulate hair growth and strength, slows down premature hair loss and graying, and heals dry, itchy scalps and dandruff. In skin care preparations, it works well on acne, tones and hydrates the skin, and can even be used as part of a cellulite treatment.

Rosewood *(Aniba rosaeodora)*: Spicy, sweet, floral aroma. Rosewood oil is an antidepressant, analgesic, antiseptic, and deodorizer. Helps with inflamed skin and scarring; great for skin care lotions and cleansers.

* *

Sage *(Salvia officinalis)*: Sharp, herbaceous scent. Sage is reputed to be anti-inflammatory; antibacterial; and helpful for increasing circulation, easing fluid retention, and soothing an upset stomach. This oil works well on acne-prone skin and is a wonderful tonic for the hair and scalp. *(Not to be confused with clary sage, which has similar characteristics to sage oil and can be used as an alternative.)*

* *

Sandalwood *(Santalum album)*: Nutty, woodsy, masculine scent. Sandalwood is known to be an antiseptic, making it a good for oily skin; however, it is also moisturizing to the skin, so it is wonderful in facial lotions. Its aromatherapy benefits are said to be antidepressant, antianxiety, and aphrodisiac.

* *

Spearmint *(Mentha spicata)*: Sweet, minty scent. Spearmint is great for relieving nausea and headaches; the aroma stimulates the mind.

* *

Sweet orange *(Citrus sinensis)*: Often referred to as just orange oil, this is a favorite oil for its uplifting, citrusy aroma. Great for use in household recipes from cleansers to room sprays. It's a great astringent and helps brighten dull skin.

* *

Tea tree *(Melaleuca alternifolia)*: Medicinal, woodsy, herbal scent. Tea tree is considered an antibiotic, antiseptic, antibacterial, and antifungal. Immune-boosting tea tree can be used on a variety of ailments, from insect bites, acne, and ringworm to sores and headaches. Great to use around the house in disinfecting cleansers and soaps.

* *

Thyme *(Thymus vulgaris)*: Herbal, clean scent. Excellent for hair care recipes, thyme helps reduce hair loss and fight dandruff. As an antifungal and antibacterial, thyme is often used to treat muscle cramps, cuts, dermatitis, insect bites, and oily skin.

* *

Turmeric *(Curcuma longa)*: Spicy, earthy, woodsy aroma. Turmeric is considered an antioxidant and anti-inflammatory, and therefore is great for arthritis care and joint and muscle aches and pains. It's also believed to be an anticancer agent. In skin care preparations, it can be beneficial in soothing

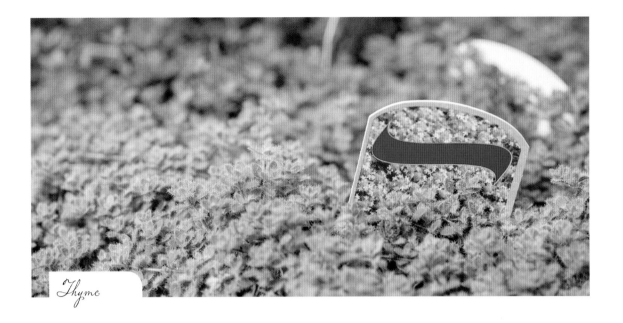

Thyme

eczema, fighting oily and acne-prone skin, reducing wrinkles, healing wounds, and lightening skin pigmentation. Great in hair care treatment oils for the prevention of hair loss.

* *

Vetiver *(Vetiveria zizanioides)*: Deep woodsy, smoky aroma. Believed to be an immune system tonic. It eases anxiety and relaxes the nerves, relieving stress and achy joints and muscles. Great in skin care recipes for balancing oil production and treating acne and sores.

* *

Ylang ylang *(Canangium odoratum)*: Floral, sweet scent. In skin care recipes, can be used to balance oil production, treat acne, fight wrinkles, and treat dermatitis. Its aroma helps aid exhaustion and treat insomnia.

↛ WHAT TO AVOID ↚

When using natural plants, it's important to research every herb prior to use. There are some herbs that may be dangerous if used incorrectly or used at all. The following is a list of essential oils that should be AVOIDED.

* Bitter almond
* Calamus
* Horseradish
* Jaborandi leaf
* Mugwort
* Pennyroyal
* Rue
* Sassafras
* Savin
* Tansy
* Thuja
* Wormseed
* Wormwood
* Yellow camphor

HERBS (DRIED OR FRESH)

When purchasing herbs, always look for organic, wild-crafted herbs. If you choose to use dried herbs over fresh, always remember to use half of what the recipe calls for, because dried herbs tend to be stronger than fresh. Often you'll find that dried herbs are easier to source and often last longer. Once you find a company you know supplies quality herbs, stick with it; searching for cheaper deals never works out.

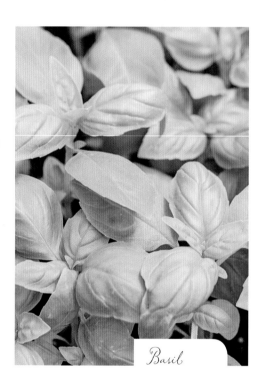

Basil

Alfalfa leaf *(Medicago sativa)*: Stimulates the appetite, aids in digestion, and is considered an anti-inflammatory. Rich in vitamins A, D, E, G, K, and P, as well as magnesium and calcium. When used in skin care, it is excellent for treating dry, itchy skin and as an astringent.

* *

Amaranth *(Amaranthus caudatus)*: A great anti-inflammatory; reduces swelling; treats dry, itchy skin, eczema, and psoriasis. Amaranth is also believed to help with stomach flu, diarrhea, and gastroenteritis.

* *

Basil *(Ocimum sanctum)*: Great for strengthening the hair, preventing hair loss, and restoring shine and manageability. It is also said to have antiaging properties.

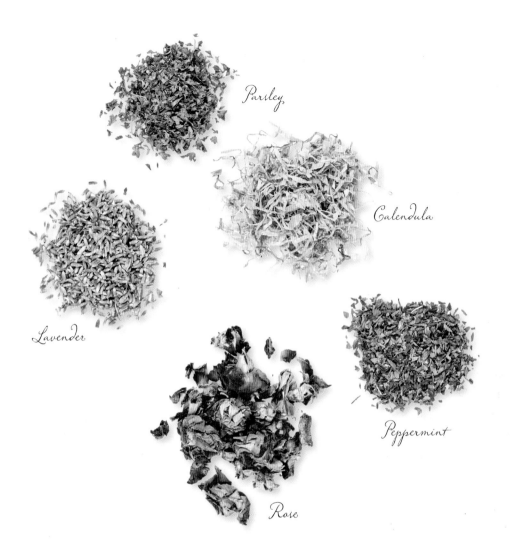

Parsley

Calendula

Lavender

Peppermint

Rose

Black pekoe tea *(Camellia sinensis)* (a.k.a. orange pekoe tea): Rich in antioxidant properties, enhances youthfulness, slows down the aging process, fights against cancer, and helps with circulatory problems.

* *

Blue malva flowers *(Malva sylvestris)*: Contains antioxidants, soothes sore throats caused by coughs and colds, and disinfects wounds. In hair care recipes it helps reduce yellowing of gray hair, and it conditions and detangles dry, coarse hair.

* *

Burdock *(Arctium lappa)*: Rich in iron, magnesium, and thiamine, this herb works wonders on the skin, treating issues such as eczema, psoriasis, sores, and acne. Great for purifying the blood, eliminating toxins, and stimulating digestion.

* Oils parents should avoid using on their infants: Basil, bay, benzoin, bergamot, birch, black pepper, cassia, citronella, clove, costus, cumin, eucalyptus, fennel, fir, ginger, helichrysum, juniper, lemon verbena, melissa, nutmeg, oak moss, orange, oregano, parsley seed, peppermint, pimento berry, pine, tagetes, thyme (red)

* Oils safe for infants: Never use essential oil neat on your infant's skin, and only use it in small quantities:
Chamomile, lavender

* Oils safe for children two months to five years old, again, never neat and in small quantities:
Chamomile, dill, eucalyptus, lavender, lemon, mandarin, tea tree

* Children five years and older can use any of the above as well as the following, again, never neat and in small quantities:
Geranium, lime, neroli, peppermint, petitgrain, rosemary, tangerine

Calendula *(Calendula officinalis)*: This herb is an antiseptic and promotes healing and cell repair. Useful for its skin-soothing properties in treating dry or irritated skin, eczema, psoriasis, sores, burns, and bruises. Used internally for fever, stomach upset, and indigestion.

* *

Chamomile *(Matricaria chamomilla)*: An antibacterial that aids in healing, rashes, abrasion burns, and irritated skin. Helps calm the nerves and ease tension.

* *

Comfrey *(Symphytum officinale)*: Commonly used as a skin treatment to stimulate cell growth and repair; also acts as an anti-inflammatory and antifungal. (Not recommended for internal use.)

* *

Clove *(Syzygium aromaticum)*: Clove is thought to be an antimicrobial, antifungal, antiseptic, and an aphrodisiac. Used to treat a variety of ailments, including toothache, indigestion, bronchial irritation, headache, and stress.

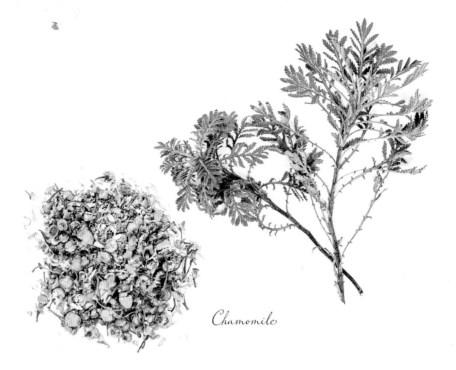

Chamomile

Dandelion root and leaves *(Taraxacum officinale)*: An amazing plant that serves as both a food and a medicine. Medicinally, dandelion stimulates liver activity, eases bowel issues, and acts as a diuretic. Because of its blood-cleansing ability, it helps eliminate toxins, treating skin irritations.

* *

Echinacea *(Echinacea angustifolia)*: Echinacea has long been used for its immune-boosting powers, preventing and defending against colds and flu. Purifies the blood and helps with such skin conditions as eczema and acne.

* *

Elder *(Sambucus nigra)*: Used to treat bronchial irritation, asthma, and allergies and to reduce fever. Its properties are similar to caffeine in that it suppresses the appetite, stimulates metabolism, and acts as a diuretic. When used in skin care preparations, it works to brighten the skin, fading dark spots.

* *

Eucalyptus *(Eucalyptus globulus)*: Known for its powerful menthol aroma, eucalyptus is often used to treat colds and congestion. It is medicinally known for its antibiotic, antibacterial properties.

* *

Fennel *(Foeniculum vulgare)*: Great in a digestive tea, fennel helps reduce flatulence and abdominal cramps, stimulates digestion, and eases colic. In nursing mothers, it stimulates breast milk production. It can also be used in toothpastes, mouthwashes, and lotions, where it helps with the appearance of aging skin.

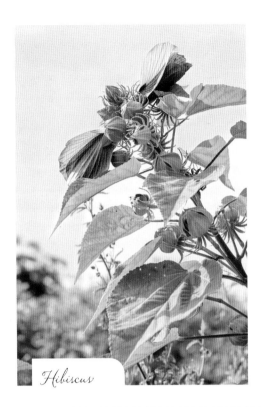
Hibiscus

Fenugreek *(Trigonella foenum-graecum)*: Soothes bronchial and throat irritations. Aids with intestinal irritations and flatulence. Stimulates lactation in nursing mothers. Fenugreek is very bitter and often needs to be mixed with other herbs or honey to be palatable.

* *

Feverfew *(Tanacetum parthenium)*: This herb functions similar to that of aspirin, relieving inflammation, swelling, menstrual cramps, and headaches.

* *

Ginger *(Zingiber officinale)*: Helps with upset stomach and relieves nausea and flatulence. Ginger also has anti-inflammatory properties, and is known to promote sweating, flushing toxins and aiding in the treatment of colds and flu. Ginger is great for bronchial irritations and sore throats.

* *

Goldenseal *(Hydrastis canadensis)*: Has anti-inflammatory, antimicrobial, and laxative properties. Good for skin care preparations for oily or acne-prone skin or to treat minor wounds and fungal infections. Goldenseal is also believed to be useful in the treatment of colds, flu, and sinus and chest congestion.

* *

Hibiscus *(Hibiscus rosa-sinensis)*: A favorite herb for the hair, hibiscus promotes hair growth, thickens the hair, eases scalp irritation, and prevents premature graying. In powder form, it has a red hue that's great for maintaining red hair. Hibiscus is beneficial for softening the skin while firming and lifting.

* *

Horsetail *(Equisetum arvense)*: A diuretic, gently stimulating increased urinary flow. Horsetail, with its high mineral content, helps heal bones and joints. Also used for the hair to treat dandruff and improve overall scalp and hair health.

* *

Juniper berries *(Juniperus communis)*: Contain tannins, flavonoids, and vitamins B and C. They are thought to improve kidney health, lower blood sugar, improve digestion, treat flatulence, ease sore joints and muscles, and expel respiratory problems. Juniper berries are considered an antimicrobial, fighting against bacteria and fungi.

* *

Lavender *(Lavandula angustifolia)*: A mild antidepressant; eases headaches, soothes an upset stomach, and relieves tension, insomnia, and stress. On the skin, lavender is soothing to insect bites, burns, minor wounds, and dryness.

* *

Lemon balm *(Melissa officinalis)*: Great when used to treat digestive problems. Lemon balm is thought to be an antidepressant; relieves stress and headaches and helps fight colds and flu.

* *

Lemon verbena *(Aloysia triphylla)*: The uplifting aroma is great for relieving stress and calming the nerves. Aids digestion, reduces nausea, and relieves bronchial and nasal congestion.

* *

Licorice *(Glycyrrhiza glabra)*: Great for the digestive system, balances female reproductive system, and helps relieve bronchial congestion, coughs, and sore throats. This herb is good for oily skin types, eczema, insect bites, burns, wounds, and skin discoloration. When used for hair care recipes, stimulates hair growth and strength.

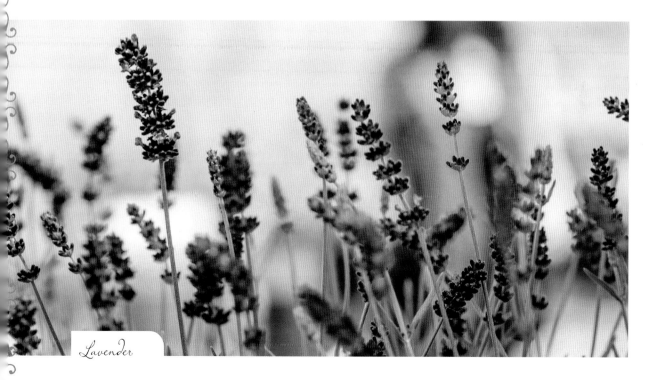

Lavender

Linden flowers *(Tilia cordata)*: Has a general sedative effect, calming the nerves and digestive system and reducing respiratory congestion. Tones and helps rid blemishes on the skin.

* *

Marshmallow *(Althaea officinalis)*: Used to treat sore throats, diarrhea, constipation, and bronchial irritation and soreness. Marshmallow is very soothing to skin irritation, and good in baths and toners meant to calm the skin.

* *

Milk thistle *(Silybum marianum)*: A powerful antioxidant that fights signs of aging and a wonderful liver tonic. Because of both of these properties, milk thistle is great for the skin to cleanse and repair.

* *

Nettle *(Urtica dioica)*: Stimulates hair growth, fights dandruff and dry scalp, eases joint pain, and cleanses the skin.

* *

Oat straw *(Avena sativa)*: Calms the nervous system. Rich in calcium and magnesium, it's great for the teeth and bones. It is also believed to act as an antidepressant and mind stimulant.

* *

Oregon grape *(Mahonia aquifolium)*: Anti-inflammatory, antiseptic, and antiviral. Very cleansing to the skin and helps soothe and treat skin conditions.

* *

Parsley *(Petroselinum crispum)*: Has diuretic properties, stimulates the appetite, and aids in digestion. Great for freshening the breath. Used in skin care to soothe irritated skin, remove blackheads, and treat bruises.

* *

Passionflower *(Passiflora incarnata)*: Soothes and supports the nerves, relaxing tension and headaches and aiding in sleep.

* *

Peppermint *(Mentha piperita)*: Great for digestion and nausea, peppermint can also be used in toothpastes and mouthwashes to freshen the breath.

Red clover *(Trifolium pratense)*: Relieves bronchial irritations and supports and relaxes the nerves. When used externally, it is great in the treatment of wounds and burns.

* *

Red raspberry *(Rubus idaeus)*: Rich in iron, niacin, and manganese, this herb increases energy levels, supports healthy joint and bone function, and promotes healthy skin and hair.

* *

Rose *(Rosa spp.)*: Rich in bioflavonoids for a healthy heart, rose soothes bronchial irritation and is uplifting and relieving to the nerves and spirit.

Yarrow

* *

Sage *(Salvia officinalis)*: A digestive tonic, congestion reliever, and sore throat soother.

* *

Valerian *(Valeriana officinalis)*: A nervous system relaxant, it eases insomnia, relieves tension, and soothes headaches and pain.

* *

Watercress *(Nasturtium officinale)*: Helps relieve bronchial irritations, colds and flu, and constipation. Also useful in relieving bad breath and treating swollen feet and ankles. Watercress is great for hair treatments to prevent hair loss, and promotes healthy hair and skin.

* *

Yarrow *(Achillea millefolium)*: Reduces fever, stimulates digestion, tones varicose veins, treats acne, and is considered an anti-inflammatory.

* *

Yellow dock *(Rumex crispus)*: Eases many skin disorders such as eczema, psoriasis, and acne. Stimulates the digestive system and liver.

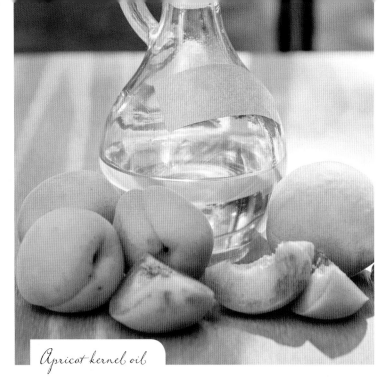

Apricot kernel oil

BUTTERS AND CARRIER OILS

Butters and carrier oils act as an essential part of all your blends. Not only do they serve as base oils for essential oil blends, but they also impart many healthful benefits. They are healing, restorative, and soothing and can be the main active ingredients in your formula. Therefore, it's essential that you do research when purchasing them. Like essential oils, some base oils and butters can be very expensive and some can be quite affordable; if a deal seems too good to be true, it often is. I always like to purchase organic.

Acai oil *(Euterpe oleracea)*: Rich in essential fatty acids, this oil is great for mature, dry skin types. It is also useful in the treatment of acne, psoriasis, and eczema.

****

Apricot kernel oil *(Prunus armeniaca)*: Vitamins A, C, and E, along with potassium, make this oil great for dry, irritated skin. Lovely in lip treatments, massage oil, and body oils.

****

Argan oil *(Argania spinosa)*: An antioxidant, antibacterial, and anti-inflammatory, this oil reduces swelling, soothes irritated skin, nourishes the hair and scalp, and has great antiaging properties.

****

Avocado oil *(Persea gratissima)*: Rich in vitamins and essential fatty acids, this oil is wonderful in the treatment of eczema, psoriasis, and scars, and is extremely hydrating to the skin and hair.

****

Baobab oil *(Adansonia digitata)*: A highly moisturizing emollient rich in vitamins A, D, E, and F. Baobab oil improves skin elasticity, encourages regeneration of skin cells, and does not clog the pores.

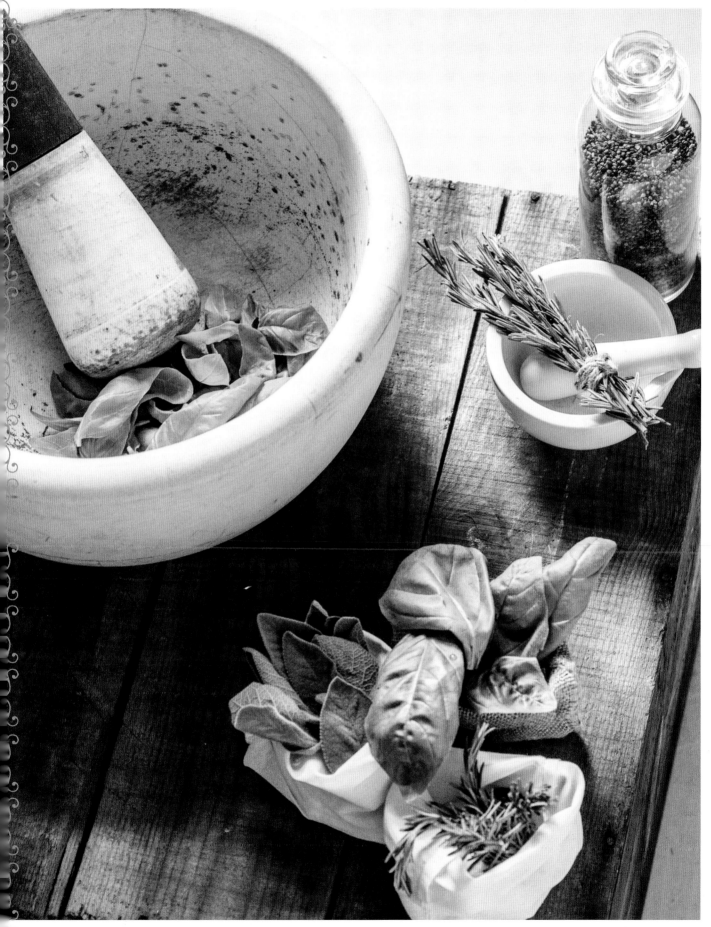

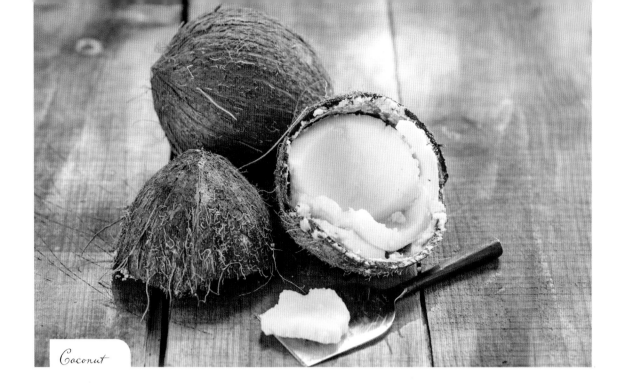

Coconut

Borage oil (*Borago officinalis*): A true skin-healing oil, borage helps in treating eczema, atopic dermatitis, and psoriasis. Borage oil is superior for restoring moisture and smoothness to overly dry or sun-damaged skin.

* *

Broccoli seed oil (*Brassica oleracea italica*): Rich in vitamin A and essential fatty acids, broccoli seed oil penetrates and hydrates the skin and doesn't leave a greasy feel. In the hair, it imparts sheen and luster.

* *

Buriti fruit oil (*Mauritia flexuosa*): Rich in essential fatty acids and carotenoids, including beta-carotene, buriti fruit oil works to treat, rebuild, hydrate, and heal the skin, especially from sun damage. Protecting the skin from free radical damage, it also possesses a natural SPF factor.

* *

Camellia oil (*Camellia oleifera*): Great for use in mature skin care recipes, this oil is full of antioxidants that block free radicals and help balance skin tone. Can also be used in hair care recipes to promote hair growth and shine.

* *

Cocoa butter (*Theobroma cacao*): This is a favorite for healing the skin, and it works well on scars, stretch marks, burns, and dry, itchy skin. It's full of natural antioxidants, so it's great for fighting the signs of aging.

Coconut oil *(Cocos nucifera)*: Exceptional oil for dry, itchy, or sensitive skin. It won't clog pores and it absorbs readily into the skin, locking in moisture.

* *

Evening primrose oil *(Oenothera biennis)*: A wonderful oil in facial lotions and serums, it helps a variety of skin types and issues, including dry, itchy skin, rosacea, acne, and mature skin.

* *

Grapeseed oil *(Vitis vinifera)*: An inexpensive but great oil, it's good for skin conditions such as dry, itchy skin, varicose veins, eczema, and psoriasis.

* *

Hazelnut oil *(Corylus americana)*: A light, penetrating oil that is slightly astringent. Great for acne-prone skin care recipes. Soothing and healing to dry, irritated skin.

* *

Jojoba oil *(Simmondsia chinensis)*: Jojoba is a great oil for any skin type or hair type. Close to our own natural oils, jojoba doesn't leave the skin oily and absorbs quickly. It's regenerative and firming and helps prevent wrinkles. Adds shine and manageability to hair and moisturizes the scalp.

Rosehips

* *

Meadowfoam seed oil *(Limnanthes alba)*: Rich in antioxidants, helps fight the signs of aging, and hydrates the skin.

* *

Neem oil *(Azadirachta indica)*: This oil possesses antibacterial, antiviral, antifungal, and antiseptic properties. Helps treat eczema, psoriasis, ringworm, and lice and controls dandruff. Great for use in moisturizers, soaps, toothpastes, and hair care products.

* *

Olive oil *(Olea europaea)*: Nourishing and calming to the skin; helps with wrinkles, brittle hair, and brittle nails.

Pumpkin seed oil *(Cucurbita pepo)*: Rich in essential fatty acids and antioxidants, this oil helps with rosacea, eczema, psoriasis, burns, wounds, and scars.

* *

Red raspberry seed oil *(Rubus idaeus)*: With high levels of essential fatty acids and the antioxidant vitamin E, this oil boasts a natural SPF of around 30 to 50. As an anti-inflammatory, it helps with dry skin, eczema, and psoriasis.

* *

Rosehip oil *(Rosa canina)*: Rich in vitamin C, rosehip smoothes and hydrates fine lines and wrinkles, repairs damaged tissue, and fades age spots.

* *

Sesame seed oil *(Sesamum indicum)*: Rich in essential fatty acids, sesame seed oil helps maintain integrity and moisturize the skin. Great choice for use in massage oil and sun care oil formulations.

* *

Shea butter *(Butyrospermum parkii)*: Both an anti-inflammatory and an antimicrobial, shea butter is used to treat extremely dry skin, burns, scars, psoriasis, eczema, dandruff, and stretch marks.

* *

Sunflower oil *(Helianthus annuus)*: Rich in both antioxidants and essential fatty acids, sunflower oil has a light texture, absorbs easily into the skin, and is soothing and softening.

* *

Sweet almond oil *(Prunus amygdalus)*: Contain vitamins A, B, and E. This oil is great for mature, dry, chapped, or inflamed skin.

* *

Watermelon seed oil *(Citrullus vulgaris)*: Rich in essential fatty acids, watermelon seed oil helps restore elasticity to the skin. This oil does not clog pores, and it works well on all skin types, from dry and mature to oily and acne-prone.

* *

Wheat germ oil *(Triticum vulgare)*: Rich in vitamins A, D, and E, wheat germ oil is very nourishing to the skin. It prevents moisture loss and soothes irritated, sunburned, or burned skin.

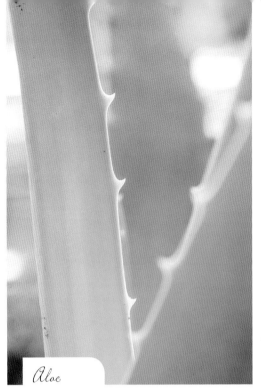

Aloe

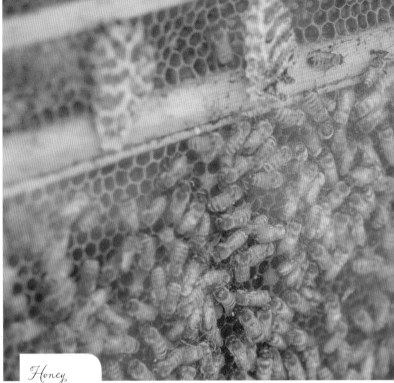

Honey

OTHER USEFUL INGREDIENTS

To create many of these recipes, you will need some additional ingredients, many of which can already be found in your kitchen.

Aloe vera gel (powder or juice): Amazing healing power. It relieves acne, soothes sunburn, prevents hair loss, and relieves dandruff. Aloe vera is quite fragile and will readily grow bacteria when contaminated. When using aloe vera gel in a formulation, you will need to properly preserve it.

* *

Almonds: Great when ground up to use in facial scrubs, they make the skin smooth and soft.

* *

Apple cider vinegar: The cure-all for some, apple cider vinegar has many health benefits. When taken internally, it cleanses the system and speeds metabolism. In hair care recipes it stimulates hair growth, adds shine, and relieves dandruff. On the skin it helps relieve eczema and psoriasis and treat acne.

* *

Arnica: Arnica oil is known for its ability to reduce inflammation and bruising.

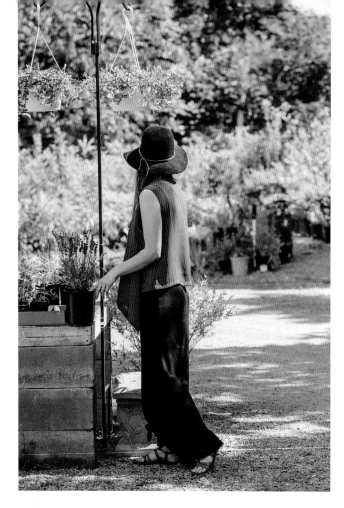

Arrowroot: A wonderful substitute for talc in body powders, arrowroot powder also gives a silky feel to water when added to a milk bath. Great to use in hair powders, body powders, baby powders, and deodorant.

* *

Baking soda: Has several uses in skin care, hair care, and household cleansing, from treating acid indigestion and heartburn to absorbing odors and cleaning teeth. Very effective in cleaning and scrubbing.

* *

Beeswax: Great when used as a thickener in recipes, beeswax is an emollient and softens the skin.

* *

Borax: Can be used in creams, lotions, shampoos, gels, and bath salts. It is an emulsifier, preservative, cleansing agent, and buffering agent.

* *

Candelilla wax: Candelilla wax is a natural vegetable wax, which is hard, brittle, slightly tacky, and usually light yellow. Used in many different products, it's often part of vegan skin care recipes as an alternative to beeswax.

* *

Coffee grounds: Helps improves circulation, acts as a diuretic, and exfoliates.

* *

Cream of tartar: Used to keep sugar syrup from crystallizing, it can also, when combined with baking soda, act as an antimicrobial and teeth whitener.

Dead Sea salt (coarse): Has the highest mineral content of all the salts, making it ideal for use in spa treatments and for bath salts and scrubs.

* *

Dulse: This red seaweed is an excellent source of phytochemicals, minerals, and iodine. Works well for treating cellulite.

* *

Emulsifying wax: Plant-based, emulsifying wax is great for its ability to bind oil and water, making it a useful ingredient when making lotions and cleansers.

→ HOW TO SOURCE INGREDIENTS ←

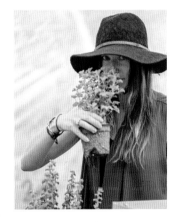

When sourcing ingredients, it is important to use reputable vendors and, as mentioned before, organic when available. Many of the ingredients in this book can be found at your local grocery store, health food store, and farmers' market. When purchasing online, use caution and do your research; if you're uncertain about a company, don't use it. There are a vast number of companies out there selling natural ingredients for medicinal and cosmetic recipes, so never settle for inferior quality and never just purchase what is cheapest; there is usually a reason. Quality and manufacturing processes should be important factors in your ingredient purchases. Also, be creative if you can't find a particular ingredient; look for a substitute or get inspiration from your nursery or farmers' market. Using what's in season means your ingredients will be healthy, fresh, and easily available. Nature provides us with many ingredients and their uses are often varied, so keep in mind that what you may purchase for your salad or soup may also double as your facial cleanser or scrub.

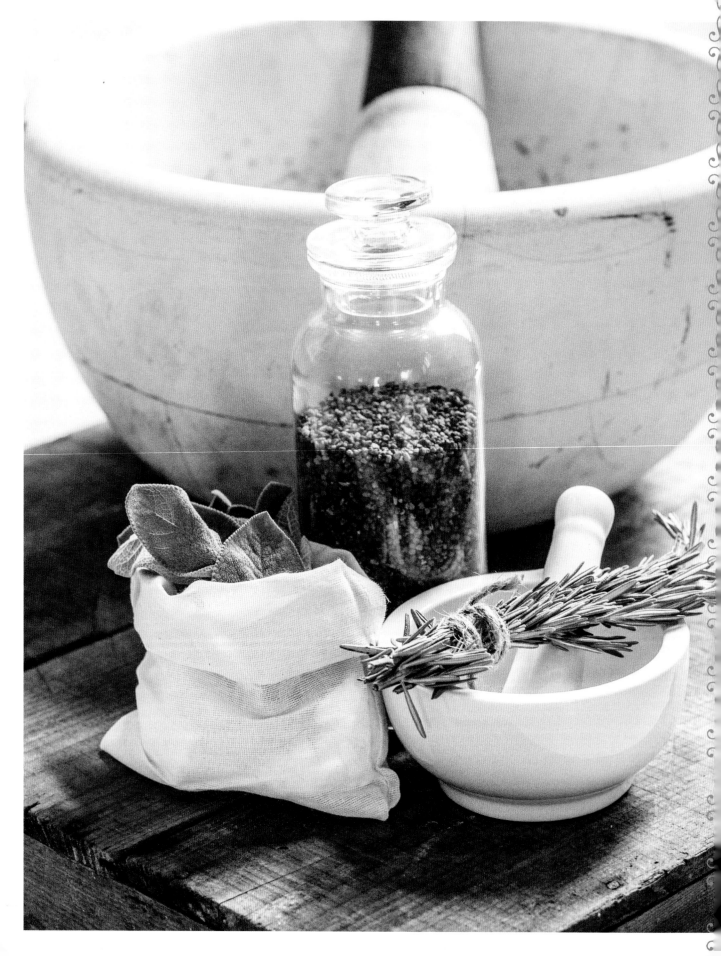

Honey: With its many uses both internal and external, honey is a must-have ingredient. Loaded with antioxidants, it reduces the risk of cancer and heart disease, treats stomach disorders, is an antibacterial and antifungal, improves energy levels, treats wounds and burns, soothes coughs and colds, and is a natural humectant. Honey can be used in teas and syrups, and can be used alone as a facial cleanser or mixed into facial recipes. Also great for the hair and as a sugar substitute.

* *

Kaolin clay: Great for use in skin care recipes. Its natural adsorbent properties make it an essential ingredient for many cosmetic recipes, from soaps, scrubs, and deodorants to facial powders and masks. Its gentleness makes it great for all skin types, even sensitive skin.

* *

Kelp powder: An underwater plant rich in vitamins and minerals. Great for use in body wraps and cellulite treatments.

* *

Pumice powder: A volcanic ash, pumice is very abrasive but also surprisingly very soft. Pumice is actually one of the softest abrasives in use today. Pumice powder is typically used in exfoliating soaps and cleansers, foot scrubs, and household cleaning recipes where you really need good scrubbing.

* *

Rhassoul clay: This reddish brown cosmetic clay from Morocco can be used in soaps, shampoos, skin conditioners, and facial masks. Great for the skin, it reduces dryness and flakiness, and improves the skin's clarity and firmness while removing impurities.

* *

Titanium oxide: Great for use as a natural sunscreen; often used in mineral makeup recipes.

* *

Witch hazel: Considered to have astringent, antiseptic, anti-inflammatory, antimicrobial, antibacterial, antifungal, and anesthetic properties, it has a variety of different medicinal and cosmetic uses.

* *

Zinc oxide: Great for use as a natural sunscreen; often used in mineral makeup recipes.

Preservatives

The recipes in this book either contain ingredients that work as natural preservatives, a recipe is only enough for a single use, or a shelf life is mentioned. Should you want to make larger batches or you just don't feel comfortable not using a preservative, the following is a brief summary of preservative use.

The first step in preserving your formulations is cleanliness. Sterilizing your work area and equipment is essential and the first line of defense against bacteria. Wearing gloves or making sure you wash your hands frequently during preparations is very important. You don't have to use harsh cleaners to sterilize your workspace; vodka or white vinegar work well. Washing your utensils in a dishwasher on high heat will work to sterilize them; for nonmetal utensil or containers, put them in the microwave for at least 2 to 3 minutes to kill bacteria and germs. Make sure your containers are clean, and avoid continually putting your fingers in your products because this is a sure way to introduce bacteria. Be sure to store your products away from sunlight and heat—or even better, keep them in the refrigerator.

There are many preservatives on the market today, with more green options coming out all the time. For at-home preparation, it is best to stick with natural preservatives. Here is a list of some natural preservatives that you can use in your cosmetic preparations. Please keep in mind that natural preservatives are not designed for unlimited storage in a warehouse, but they will serve their purpose for kitchen chemists.

Aspen bark extract: Derived from the bark of the American aspen, this bark is rich in salicylates, which inhibit the growth of mold, yeast, and *E. coli*. It should be used at a concentration of 0.2 to 3.0 percent.

* *

Essential oils: Essential oils considered to have preservative benefits include thyme, sweet orange, lemongrass, clove, eucalyptus, peppermint, and rose geranium. For most formulations, use 1 percent or less in a carrier oil.

* *

Geogard: Geogard uses naturally occurring sugar and salt to protect against bacteria. This preservative is permitted by Ecocert and NATRUE, two organizations that have developed standards and certification for organic and natural cosmetic products. Use at a concentration of 0.8 to 1.5 percent.

* *

Grapefruit extract (*Citrus grandis*)**:** This antimicrobial citrus oil is often blended with vegetable glycerin to avoid irritating the skin. Use grapefruit extract at a concentration of 0.5 to 1 percent.

Neem oil: Neem is a remarkable oil. It is antifungal, antibacterial, antiprotozoan, and a spermicide. Use at a concentration of 0.03 to 6.0 percent.

* *

Potassium sorbate: This results from a reaction of sorbic acid (a natural fatty acid) and potassium hydroxide. Used in both food and cosmetic preparations, it is active against molds and yeasts. It can be used at a concentration of 0.15 to 0.3 percent.

* *

Radish root ferment: This is active against most bacteria; it even fights against some yeasts and fungi. Use it at a concentration of 0.5 to 2.5 percent.

* *

Rosemary extract *(Rosmarinus officinalis)*: This extract is a natural preservative and antioxidant. Use undiluted rosemary extract at a concentration of 0.15 to 0.5 percent.

* *

Vitamin E *(tocopherol)*: A natural antioxidant, tocopherol, a component of vitamin E, is a great antioxidant for protecting cosmetic formulations. Use at a concentration of 0.5 to 0.8 percent.

→ A WORD OF CAUTION ←

There are a few things to consider before crafting the recipes in this book or coming up with your own. Just because it's natural doesn't mean it's not an allergen. Just as with commercial products, you can have an allergic reaction to naturals. If you have known sensitivities or not, it is always smart to do a spot test first to test for allergies. Always wait at least 24 to 48 hours after doing a spot test before applying the product. Should you have a known allergy to a natural, you can substitute something else (check the back of the book for a table of substitutions). Also, these recipes are not intended to replace a health care professional's advice and have not been approved by the FDA to treat or heal. Always check with your physician before changing any course of treatment.

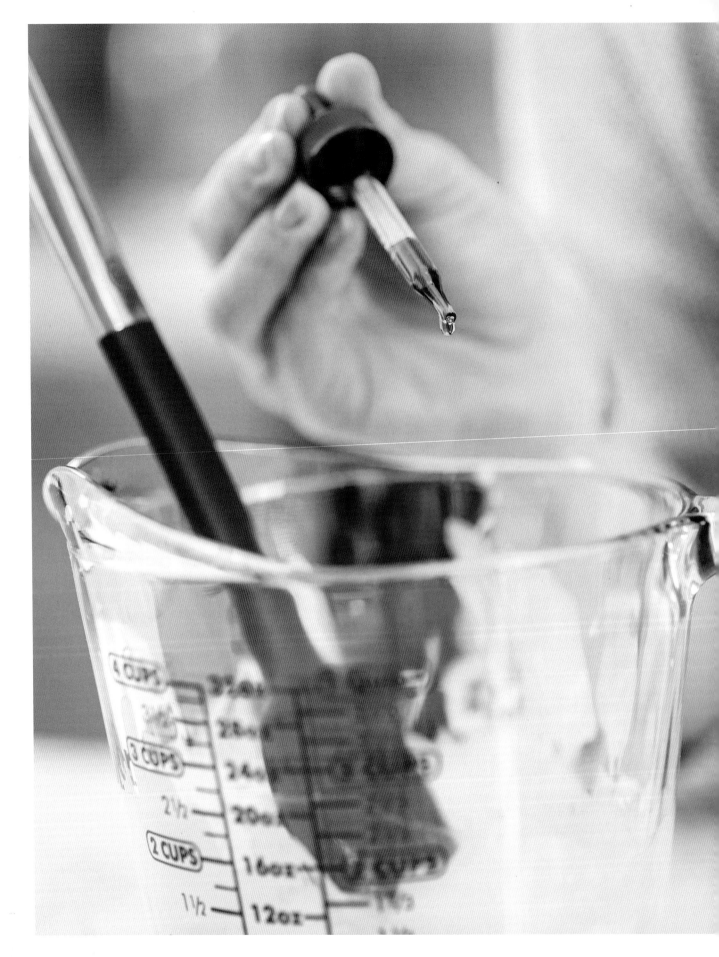

CHAPTER 3

Master the Apothecary Basics

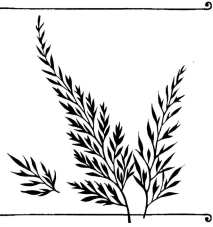

THE APOTHECARY CRAFT CONSISTS OF A SET OF SKILLS THAT TAKES YOUR HERBS, BUTTERS, AND OILS FROM THEIR NATURAL STATE AND TRANSFORMS THEM INTO TINCTURES THAT HEAL, OINTMENTS THAT SOOTHE, AND LOTIONS THAT BEAUTIFY. THIS CHAPTER WILL TEACH YOU HOW TO PREPARE YOUR NATURALS, ALLOWING YOU TO FORMULATE BOUNDLESS CREATIONS.

THE APOTHECARY TOOLBOX

Now that you've gathered your ingredients, you need to get your toolbox together. Most of the tools used to prepare the recipes in this book or ones that you'll create on your own can be found in your kitchen. However, if possible, purchase separate tools to use for your creations; this limits the possibility of contamination. Here are some of the basics you'll want to have on hand:

Coffee grinder: This will come in handy for many different recipes; a food processor or blender can also be used.

Cutting board: This is for cutting herbs and hard waxes.

Funnel: You'll need this for pouring your finished products into containers.

Measuring cups and spoons: You'll need these to measure ingredients for the recipes.

Mixing bowls: They can be metal, glass, or plastic. It's best to use glass because it can be disinfected easily (better than plastic), and metal can sometimes interact with different oils.

Mixing spoons and whisk: A selection of different spoons and stirrers in different sizes will prove to be very useful. Stainless steel is best, and for less viscous recipes, glass stirring rods are best and easily disinfected.

Mortar and pestle: You'll use these for preparing poultices.

Scale: You'll need this for measuring your ingredients, especially herbs. Most recipes in this book are measured by tablespoons and cups; as you begin to experiment, you'll find most recipes are also in grams.

Spatula: A good spatula will ensure that you get to use every last bit of your creation.

Strainers: It's best to have a few sizes of strainers for different uses. Alternatives to strainers can be cheesecloth or coffee filters.

Here are some other useful supplies:

Bottles and other containers: You will need a variety of bottles and containers. It is best to use glass containers because they can be easily cleaned and sterilized. You can easily reuse bottles; after cleaning them out, boil them or place them in the microwave for quick disinfecting.

Double boiler: This is necessary to avoid burning delicate oils and butters, but you can just as easily put a smaller pot inside a larger one in a pinch.

Eyedroppers: You will need these for measuring your essential oils. Some essential oils can be purchased with the dropper as part of the packaging.

Gloves: This is a good idea to help avoid contaminating your products.

Hand mixer: In most cases, spoons and spatulas will work fine, but sometimes it's just easier to use a hand mixer.

Knives: For cutting herbs and hard waxes or when making lozenges.

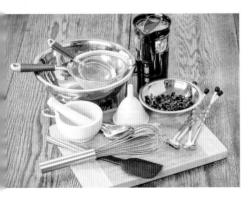
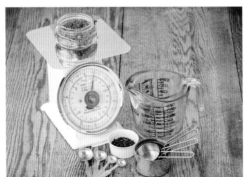
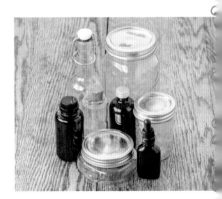

PREPARATION TECHNIQUES

In this section, you'll learn the basic techniques of the apothecary. You'll use these techniques to make the recipes in this book and more.

★ HERBAL INFUSIONS ★

There are various ways, both internal and external, for herbs to be absorbed into the body. One of these methods is herbal infusions, the most common of which are teas. Herbal infusions are made from the leaves, flowers, and aromatic parts of the plant. They should be steeped, usually in hot water; it's best not to bring the water to a boil, but rather to a simmer, because these delicate parts of the plant can lose some of their medicinal properties when boiled. For heat-sensitive herbs, you can use cold water; just allow them to steep longer. An herbal infusion or tea can be stored for up to 3 to 4 days in the refrigerator. Water isn't the only carrier used in herbal infusions; oils can also be used and are prepared in much the same way a water infusion is.

There are three different methods for preparing an infusion, depending on the plant used: simmering, cold infused, and sun infused. The infusions can be used in a variety of ways, including in beverages as drink mixers, or straight as hot or cold teas. They can also be used to make healing ointments, in perfumes and cosmetic lotions, and in cleansers. They are even used for cooking and baking. And you will see them used throughout this book for numerous recipes.

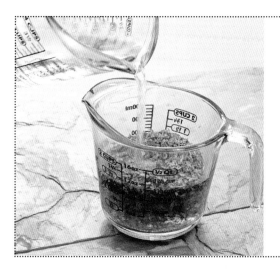

To make an herbal infusion, begin by measuring out your herbs; a general measurement guideline is 1 quart (1 L) of water per 1 to 2 ounces (28 to 56 g) of fresh herbs, but this can vary depending on the herb (for a single serving, use 1 cup [235 ml] of water per ½ tablespoon of herbs). Pour simmering water over the herbs and let them steep for 15 to 25 minutes. You should cover them while steeping to make sure you don't lose any of the plant's goodness.

You'll find that some herbs are stronger than others and steeping time can cause variations in strength. So as you experiment more, keep a log of your recipes and let your taste preferences be your guide.

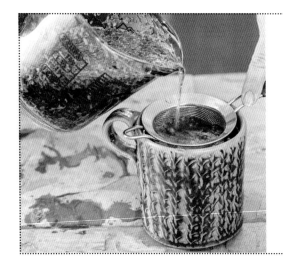

Place a strainer and cheesecloth over your cup or sealable container, strain, and enjoy.

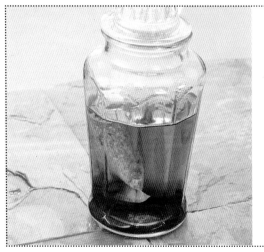

Alternatively, you can you can use a heat-sealable tea bag and pour the water directly into your container. Once you've mastered your tea blends, you can make multiple tea bags for travel or when you're in a rush. They even make great gifts for friends and family. You can purchase sealable tea bags at most health food stores and on the Web.

★ Decoctions ★

Decoctions are similar to herbal infusions; however, this method is used when you are preparing tougher parts of plants, such as wood, bark, chips, and roots. When preparing these plant types, you need to use more heat and a longer steeping time. Ideally, creating a steady simmer for a long period of time, even overnight, works best rather than bringing the water to a complete boil; this ensures the release of all the plant's constituents without losing or damaging them.

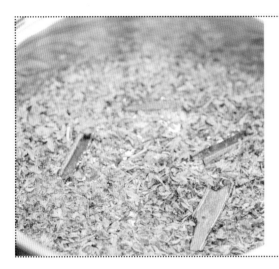

Using the same measurements as for the herbal infusion, bring water with herbs to a steady simmer and cover. Let it simmer for at least 45 minutes or longer, depending on the plant type.

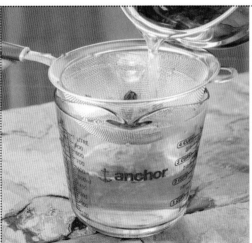

Once the allotted time has passed, place a strainer over a clean container and pour. Use the back of a spoon to press any remaining liquid through the strainer. You can use cheesecloth in place of the strainer, but be sure to wring it out. Your decoction is ready for consumption or can be stored for later use in the refrigerator for 3 to 4 days.

✴ TINCTURES ✴

Tinctures are a more concentrated form of herbal extractions. They are often made with alcohol, usually brandy or vodka, as the solvent; however, there are those who might prefer to use apple cider vinegar or vegetable glycerin as the solvent for various reasons. Often an alcohol tincture is strongest, but all methods result in a very concentrated dosage of the herb and therefore should be administered with care. Dosages are measured in drops. A standard dose for adults could be 1 to 2 drops of tincture for 5 pounds (2.2 kg) of body weight. Different plant blends can require different dosages. Dosage will also depend of the type of ailment you are treating and whether it is chronic or acute; for a more acute condition, the dosage may be smaller but more frequent. There are a ton of tincture dosage calculators available for free online and once you start creating your own blends, it's recommended that you try using them; they are a handy resource. Tinctures are almost always diluted in some type of carrier, such as water or juice, but can be taken directly on or under the tongue.

Tinctures have a long shelf life (up to 2 years or more) because the alcohol or vinegar acts as a natural preservative. You should be sure to research the plant (or plants) you intend to use in your tincture to be sure of the amount needed. Keep in mind the higher the proof alcohol, the stronger extraction it will produce. For fresh herbs, use 1 part herb to 2 parts liquid (for dried herbs increase the liquid to 5 parts). An 80-proof alcohol is usually best for tinctures; anything stronger and it may require the addition of some water to ensure the proper extraction of water-soluble parts of the herb and to avoid damaging the herb's constitutes. In this case you may also need to add more fresh herbs, from 2 parts to 3 or 4 parts. Generally, 15 to 25 percent alcohol will produce the best tincture, ensuring its curative benefits while avoiding contamination from mold. When making glycerin-based tinctures, it's best to keep the ratio at 25 percent. The addition of water will be necessary, but too much water can increase the risk of spoilage, so for every 2 parts glycerin, only ½ to 1 part water should be added. Glycerin-based tinctures are then made the same way as alcohol- or vinegar-based ones.

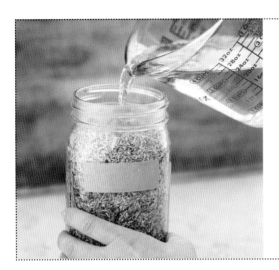

Start by gathering clean, fresh herbs or organic wild-crafted dried herbs. If you are using fresh herbs, make sure they are clean and any damaged or dying bits are removed. Then chop them; this helps with solvent penetration and will speed the process. Once you've prepared your herbs, select which solvent you will use and measure out the proper ratios. Place the herbs in a sterile sealable container, leaving about 1 inch (2.5 cm) or so of space at the top. Pour your solvent over the herbs, covering them completely.

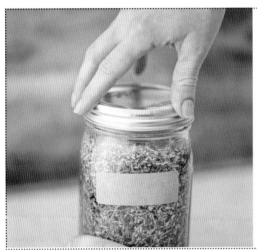

Seal the mixture tightly, give it a shake, and place it in a dark storage area, away from direct sunlight and heat (the kitchen cupboard is fine). It's also wise to label your tincture and include the date. Let the mixture macerate for at least 2 weeks or up to a month, shaking periodically.

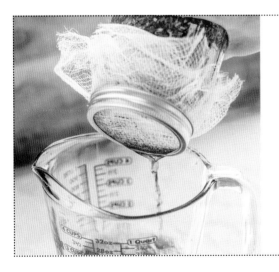

The next step is straining. Place cheesecloth or a mesh strainer over your container and strain all the liquid into a clean container. If you use cheesecloth, pour the herbs onto the cheesecloth and wring it out, making sure you get all the liquid. If you use a mesh strainer, be sure to use the back of a spoon to firmly press out any remaining liquid. Once you have strained all your liquid, pour it into a dark-colored sterile bottle, label it, and date it. An amber dropper bottle works best, for both dosage convenience and shelf life.

* Syrups *

Syrups are great alternatives to tinctures, especially for herbs with a harsher taste. This method is great to use with children or those who prefer not to use alcohol, because it has the sweetness of sugar or honey to mask the flavor of the herb. This is also a great method for throat and cough remedies, because the syrup acts to slightly coat the throat (see chapter 5 for recipes). Syrups can be made with organic sugar, honey, maple syrup, rice syrup, or other sweeteners of your choice. *Please note that it is advised by the Centers for Disease Control not to give children under the age of one raw honey due to the risk of botulism spores.*

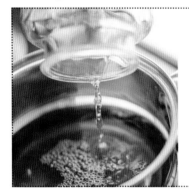

Begin by preparing an herbal infusion of your choice (see page 53). Pour the infusion into a saucepan or double boiler, and bring it to a simmer. Keep it simmering until the liquid is reduced by about half.

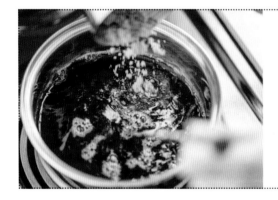

Add sweetener, which also acts as a preservative; for the basic infusion ratio of 1 quart (1 L) of water to 1 or 2 ounces (28 to 56 g) of fresh herbs, you should add 24 ounces (720 g) of organic sugar or 24 fluid ounces (720 g) of honey, stirring until the sweetener has dissolved.

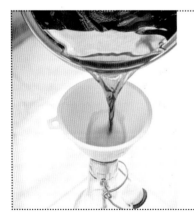

Pour the syrup into a sterilized container and seal it. Allow it to cool before using it. Label and date the bottle and store it in an area away from direct sunlight. Syrups will keep, if not contaminated, for up to 1 to 2 years.

★ Herbal Honeys ★

Honey is a powerful medicinal. Raw honey contains antibacterial enzymes. It works well when applied directly to cuts, burns, and sores. It's beneficial to the intestinal tract, provides energy, and boosts the immune system. A kitchen staple during cold season due to its antimicrobial effects, it works wonders on its own with lemon and warm water or in a medicinal recipe for coughs and sore throats (see chapter 5 for recipes). *Please note that it is advised by the Centers for Disease Control not to give children under the age of one raw honey due to the risk of botulism spores.*

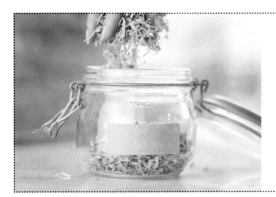

To make an herbal honey, start by selecting your herbs. When you are using fresh herbs, make sure they are clean, and then coarsely chop them. Use equal parts honey to herbs (or half the amount of herbs if using dried). This process can also be used with tinctures; use equal parts honey to tincture. Place the herbs in a sterile, sealable container.

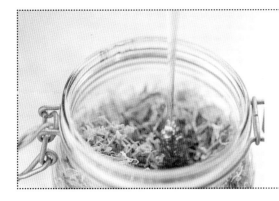

It's often easiest to work with warm honey, because it helps to release the herbs' curative properties, but be careful not to overheat or boil it. Pour the warm honey over the herbs or tincture and slowly stir the mixture.

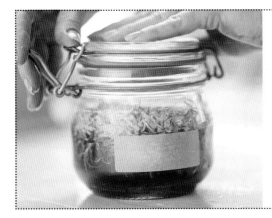

Tightly seal the jar, label it, and date it. Let the mixture macerate for at least 1 week; up to or more than a month is best. When you open for the first time, stir well before using.

★ Salves (Ointments) ★

Salves are great external medicinals (see chapter 5 for recipes). Storing a few salve blends in the refrigerator or medicine cabinet not only ensures a cure for all that ails you, from skin problems to sore muscles, but also saves you a trip to the pharmacy. Salves are easy to make, and when properly stored can last for up to 2 years. They can be made using fresh or dried herbs, and the measurements depend on how strong or gentle you prefer the end result. Apply the salve to the affected area as often as needed, or 2 to 4 times daily.

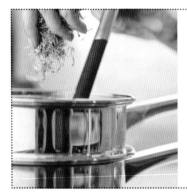

In a double boiler, heat 1 cup (235 ml) of oil, add ¼ cup (54 g) of beeswax, and melt it. Oils that can be used may depend on the desired use, but olive oil is usually preferred when preparing medicinal salves.

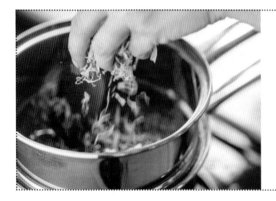

Slowly stir in the herb of your choice; a fair amount of the herb is recommended. Let it macerate over low heat for a couple of hours. Using a double boiler keeps your oils and herbs from burning, but keep an eye on the water level, as it will evaporate quickly.

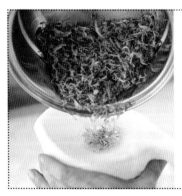

Remove from the heat. Place a cheesecloth or muslin over a clean container and pour the mixture into it.

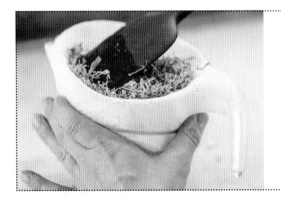

Use a spatula or the back of a large spoon to press the herbs and get any liquid out.

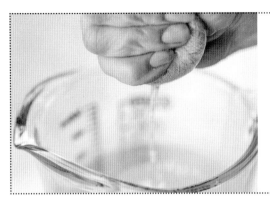

Pull the sides of the cheesecloth together, then wring out any remaining oils.

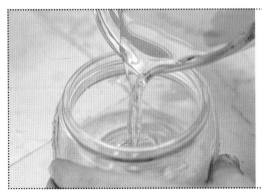

Pour into a clean, sealable container.

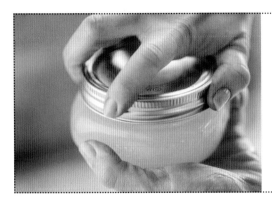

Seal, label, and date. Let stand until the ointment is cool and has solidified before use.

★ LOTIONS AND CLEANSERS ★

There are quite a few recipes in this book that require you to make either a lotion or a cleanser by heating and cooling the ingredients. Although not all skin care recipes require this method, it is usually used for more complex recipes and is essential to any cosmetic crafter. While beginner's luck is not uncommon, don't get discouraged if your first attempts do not yield the perfect emulsion.

To start, it is essential that you use sterilized equipment, utensils, and containers. Even if you are preparing your mixtures at home for your personal use only, sterilization is still important. This is true for any technique in this book; a clean work area is essential to ensuring the longest shelf life for your home preparations.

Making a lotion or lotion-based cleanser usually consists of the following: a water phase, an oil phase in which emulsifiers are added, and a cool phase, during which delicate or temperature-specific essentials are added. There are also recipes that call for only two phases, such as an oil phase to heat and melt, and then a cool phase to add the active ingredients.

The water phase should always start with distilled water; using tap water only opens the door to contamination. For the oil phase, there are many possible oils, both vegetable and nut, available for use. Make sure that, as with all other preparations, the oils you choose are fresh; organic is preferred, and refined cold-pressed oils are often recommended. Refined oils have longer shelf lives and can withstand oxidation better. Unrefined oils, while great for cooking because they are highly flavorful, have a much shorter shelf life, so it's best to leave them for cooking dinner. Be sure to store your finished products in airtight, dark, sterile containers away from sunlight.

Here I present the basics of making lotion. As you get more knowledgeable and adventurous, you can start to formulate your own recipes from scratch, which will require a little more knowledge of chemistry, such as hydrophilic-lipophilic balance (HLB), to master the technique. But for now, getting the basics is the best starting point (see chapter 4 for recipes).

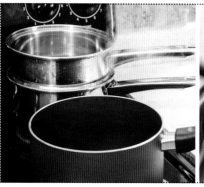
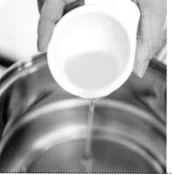

Measure out all the ingredients for phase A (water phase) and put them into a regular saucepan. Measure out all the ingredients for phase B (oil phase) and put them into a double boiler. A double boiler is used for the oils to avoid burning them.

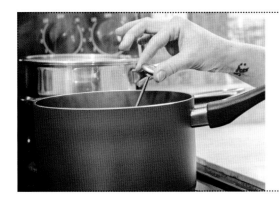

Bring both phases to 170°F (77°C).

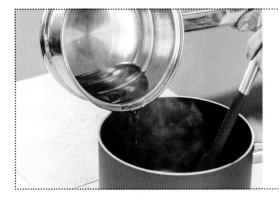

Once both phases are at the correct temperature, remove them from the heat and pour phase A into phase B, mixing continuously. Keep stirring the two phases while they start to cool.

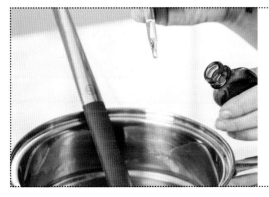

Let them cool to at least 120°F (49°C) before you add phase C. Stirring constantly, slowly mix in the phase C ingredients one at a time until completely incorporated.

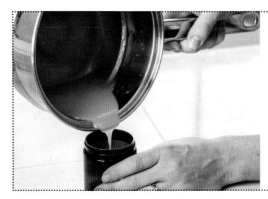

Once cooled, pour the mixture into a sterilized container, label it, and date it.

PART 2

The Apothecary's Remedies and Recipes

*

The tips and recipes in the following chapters will pamper your body both inside and out. Whether you are looking for a cure for your sore throat or the zit that won't go away, you'll find the remedy here. These recipes are great starting points for the naturals novice as well as the expert. Once you get the basics, feel free to create and adapt any of the recipes to your preferences.

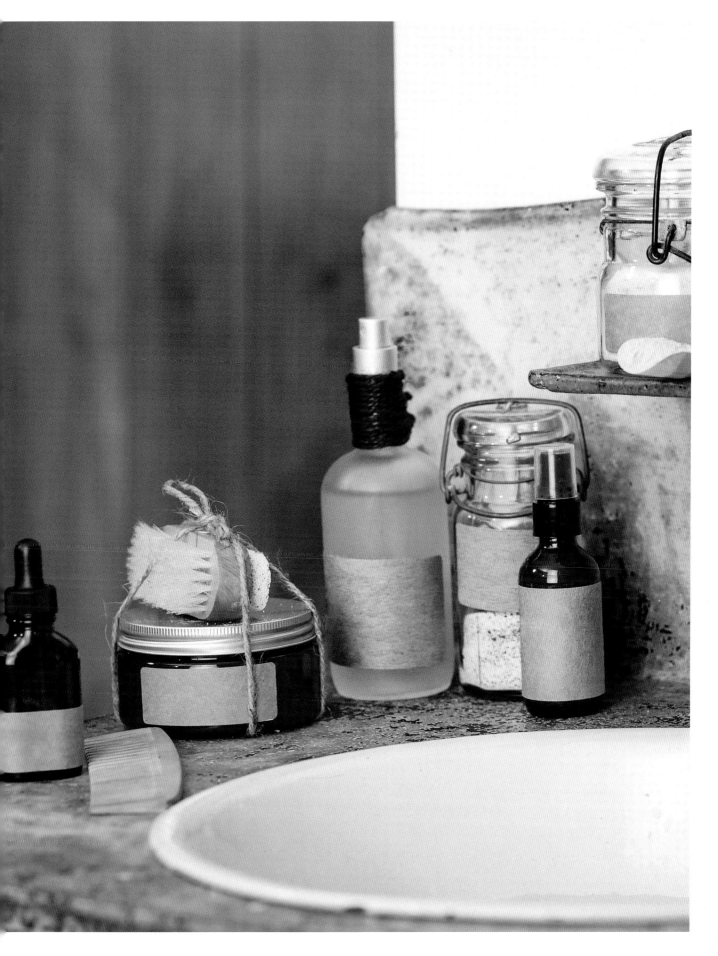

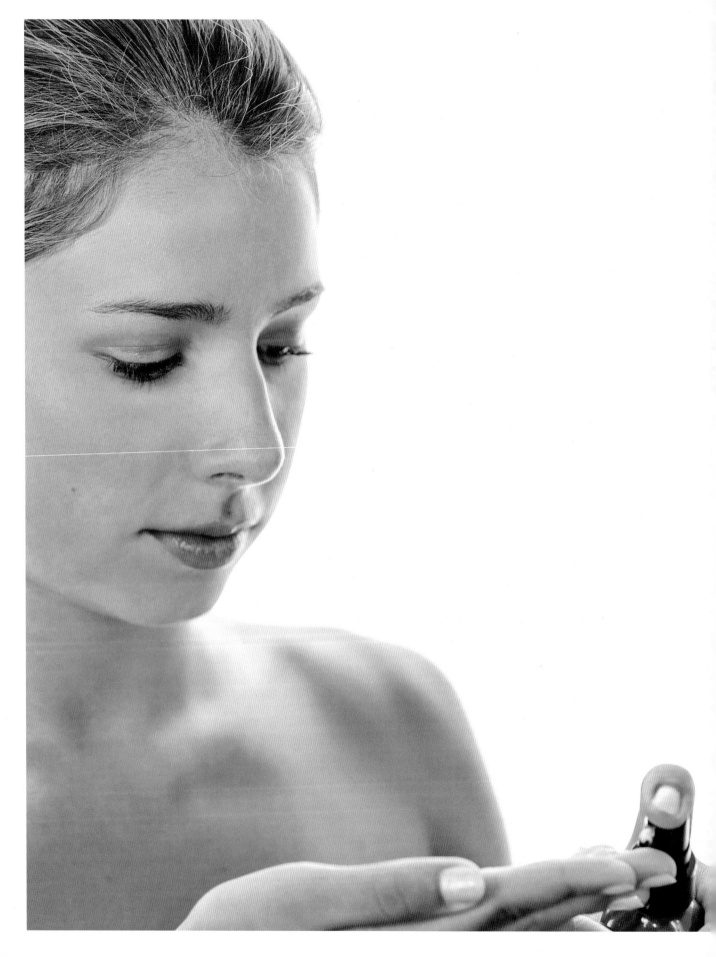

CHAPTER 4

Skin Care Recipes

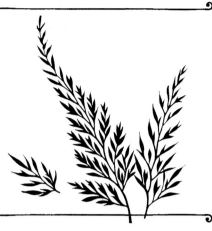

YOUR SKIN IS YOUR LARGEST ORGAN AND ABSORBS 60 PERCENT OF WHAT YOU PUT ON IT, SO LET'S STOP TAKING IT FOR GRANTED. THIS MEANS TAKING CARE OF IT ON A DAILY BASIS. THIS CHAPTER WILL TEACH YOU THE ESSENTIALS OF A DAILY SKIN CARE ROUTINE AND HOW TO MAKE ALL THE PRODUCTS THAT YOU'LL NEED FOR HAPPY, HEALTHY SKIN.

SKIN CARE 101

The tips below are the core essentials to proper skin and body well being. Always keep in mind that what you put on your body is just as important as what you put in it.

Sleep: Get plenty of sleep, and your eyes and skin will thank you. Just as the mind needs sleep to decompress itself and rejuvenate, so does the skin. The skin detoxifies and replenishes while you sleep.

* *

Exercise regularly: Exercise not only heals the body, but the mind as well. By lowering hormone levels, flushing out toxins, and boosting collagen production, exercise is vital to both body and skin health.

* *

Eat right: Consume plenty of vegetables and fruits, and limit your salt, dairy, and sugar intake. Make sure your diet consists of plenty of nutrient-rich foods that contain vitamins, minerals, and anti-oxidants (vitamins A, C, and E), not processed, empty-calorie, sugary foods. One nutrient especially good for the skin is biotin (a B vitamin), which helps replenish not only the skin but the hair and nails as well. Although there are plenty of supplements out there, nothing is as good as getting your nutrients from your food. Plenty of greens, fruits, and healthy proteins are essential for a healthy glow.

* *

Restrict caffeine intake: Reduce your caffeine intake as much as possible. Try to avoid other bad habits, such as smoking and drinking alcohol. All of these dehydrate the skin and increase wrinkles. If you must have coffee, instead of two cups of coffee try switching that second cup to green tea if you really need the extra caffeine. Herbal teas are great morning pick-me-ups sans the effects of caffeine.

* *

Drink plenty of water: What you put in your body directly affects what's on the outside. Hydrate, hydrate, and hydrate, if you truly want great skin. Drinking plenty of water or healthy, sugar-free, chemical-free fluids helps flush the system of toxins and keeps the skin moist and plump.

* *

Relax: Often easier said than done! Try to find activities that calm you: read a book, take a yoga class, or do some breathing exercises. If you calm the body, the skin will be calm as well.

* *

Keep your skin clean: Follow a healthy skin care regimen and your skin will thank you. Start with cleansing your face in the morning and at night. Find or make yourself a cleanser that works well for your skin type. Follow that with a toner and then a moisturizer to benefit and balance your particular skin type. Once a week you should do a facial mask and also exfoliate. Exfoliating shouldn't stop with your face; your body will benefit greatly from a healthy scrub. Not only should you avoid skin care products laden with harmful chemicals, but also keep in mind that our skin absorbs 60 percent of everything we put on it. This includes things the environment puts on it as well. The toxins in our environment are absorbed through our skin and bacteria and oils build up all day, so it is important to keep the skin clean. Washing in the morning rids the skin of the toxins our bodies have flushed out while we slept. Also, changing your pillowcase often is a very good idea. Toners often add a further astringent, cleansing action, nourishing and helping to regulate pH while calming the skin. Moisturizers are essential to keeping the skin healthy; every time you wash, you should always follow with a moisturizer to replace the oils you may have stripped. The more moisturized the skin, the less oils your body will naturally produce.

* *

Enjoy the shade: Limit your sun exposure, and when you are in the sun, be sure to wear a natural SPF. People often only think of this during the summer, but winter can expose you to sun damage, too. I switched long ago to using a mineral-based foundation that naturally provides sun protection, and I try to moisturize with oils that naturally contain sun protection. If you do spend a long period of time in the sun, be sure to always give yourself a moisturizing and soothing mask afterward (an aloe or a milk mask is best for this).

★ WHAT'S YOUR SKIN TYPE? ★

In my experience, no one has one particular skin type. Most individuals have a combination of one or more skin types or so-called conditions. And this combination often changes throughout the years, or even from month to month. When choosing skin care regimens, I always recommend working from the inside out. Start by analyzing your diet: are there certain foods that you notice your skin reacts to? Are you particularly sensitive to hormone fluctuations? Do you react strongly to stress?

This chapter contains recipes that are either tailored to a particular skin type or that can be altered to be. I never use one particular skin cleanser or moisturizer, because my skin often fluctuates. I like to start with a solid, good-for-the-skin base that I can customize as needed. Feel free to experiment with the recipes and research even more base oils, herbs, and essential oils that are good for your particular skin type or the condition you may be suffering from at the time.

"Normal skin" would, by the book, be described as neither particularly dry nor oily. Normal skin types are not prone to breakouts and/or blackheads, and the skin is well balanced overall. I have yet to meet a person, female or male, who doesn't have some type of complaint about his or her skin or who claims to truly have normal skin. I'm sure they are out there, and if it's you, well, then, you're very lucky. However, the large majority of us will have at least one of the following three complaints about our skin.

MY SKIN IS OILY: The pores are enlarged, and overactive glands make your skin look oily even shortly after cleansing. You're often prone to breakouts and blackheads.

MY SKIN IS DRY: Dry skin is often, as a result, prone to fine lines and wrinkles. Dry skin can be irritated and flaky, and most often those with extremely overly dry skin suffer from eczema or psoriasis. Dry skin can also be very sensitive skin.

MY SKIN IS SENSITIVE: It has been my experience that those with sensitive skin can have either dry or oily skin, too. And most sensitive skin, if not caused by an underlying skin condition such as eczema or dermatitis, is the result of an allergy to the many synthetic harmful chemicals that are in our products. I always advise those complaining of sensitive skin to first start using naturals and then go fragrance-free. Keep in mind that even naturals can cause skin allergies, so if you are using naturals and still suffering from sensitive or irritated skin, try starting with a natural base cream (choose your naturals wisely) and then add active ingredients one by one until you can determine your trigger. I often get people who tell me they can't use products that are scented, even those scented with pure essential oils. This is often an incorrect assumption that comes from the vast number of synthetic fragrances in products that are extremely irritating to the skin. Unfortunately, cosmetic companies often label a product as "lavender scented," but the scent is far from the actual essential oil. If scents are a concern for you, start with an unscented base and then test pure essentials to determine your allergy. Patch testing any new product is always a good recommendation if you have sensitive skin. It's important to educate yourself about what you're putting on your skin. There will always be times when we don't use naturals, and I'm not telling you to go throw away every bottle in your bathroom (although I'll bet the more you learn the more you will throw out!), but please become aware of what's in them. Know what is good for you and what is harmful.

Here is a quick recipe reference of some herbs and essential oils that are great for each skin type.

Skin Type	Dry and/or Mature Skin	Sensitive Skin	Oily or Combination Skin
Carrier Oil	Sweet almond, acai, argan, borage, camellia, evening primrose, rosehip, apricot	Jojoba, sweet almond	Neem, baobab, argan, camellia, evening primrose, grapeseed, jojoba, carrot seed
Essential Oil/Extract	Chamomile, calendula, fennel, rose, lavender, patchouli, jasmine, rose, ylang ylang, geranium, palmarosa, sandalwood, vetiver, frankincense, helichrysum, everlasting, rosewood, clary sage	Lavender, chamomile, neroli, rose, vetiver, jasmine, mandarin	Licorice root, fennel, patchouli, tea tree, turmeric oil, rosemary, sage, comfrey, goldenseal, myrrh, lemongrass, petitgrain, ylang ylang, geranium, cedarwood, sandalwood, cypress, rosewood, thyme
Herb	Chamomile, alfalfa, calendula, fennel seed, comfrey	Lavender, chamomile, lemon balm, calendula	Fennel seed, tea tree leaves, turmeric powder, comfrey, sage, goldenseal

→ KITCHEN RESCUES ←

Here are some quick rescues that you'll find in your kitchen:

* **An egg and 2 tablespoons (16 g) cornstarch:** Firms the skin; apply it like a mask and leave it on for 20 minutes.

* **Cantaloupe:** Soothes dry skin; create a mash using fresh, ripe cantaloupe and rub it onto your face. Leave it on for 5 to 10 minutes before rinsing.

* **Fresh pineapple and/or papaya juice:** Natural skin whiteners; apply with a cotton ball and let it sit on the skin for at least 10 minutes before rinsing.

* **Green tea bags:** Reduces puffiness around the eyes; place dampened tea bags on eyes for 10 to 20 minutes.

* **Honey:** A natural humectant; use as a cleanser or add to almost any skin care recipe. Use it as a wetting agent for clay and powder cleansers, or add some lemon juice for oily skin or milk for dry skin.

* **Potato or cucumber slices:** Reduces puffiness and dark circles around the eyes; place cool slices on eyes for 10 to 20 minutes.

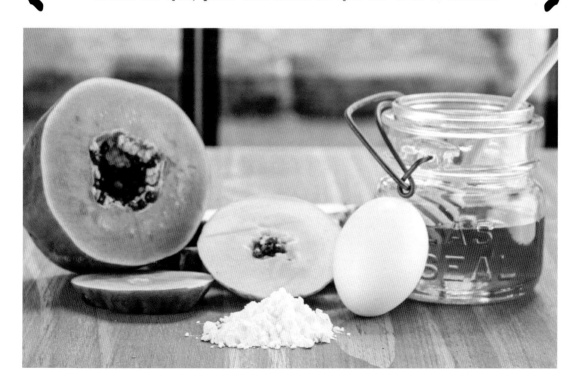

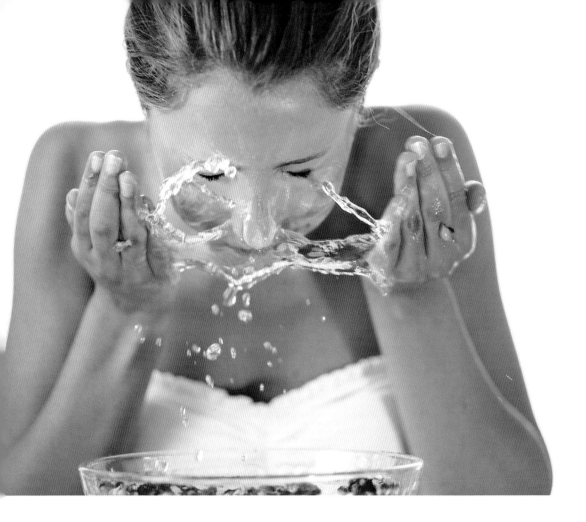

CLEANSERS AND SCRUBS

These are great cleansers to start with: they require no heating and are simple to make. The oils act not only to remove makeup and residue, but also to condition and heal. They make wonderful everyday cleansers. I love to start them on a Sunday morning and make enough for the week. These cleansers are made using the herbal infusion method described in chapter 3 (see page 53).

★ LIQUID CLEANSERS ★

You'll find that because many of these cleansers contain both water and oil, there will be separation, something that happens with most naturals. This is normal, and a quick shake prior to application is all it takes to remedy that.

⇥ ESSENTIAL OILS FOR COMMON SKIN CONDITIONS ⇤

★ **Cold sores and herpes:** Bergamot, chamomile, lemon, lavender, geranium

★ **Damaged skin:** Chamomile, lavender, sandalwood, rose, palmarosa

★ **Eczema and psoriasis:** Sandalwood, patchouli, helichrysum, palmarosa, chamomile, cedarwood, frankincense, jasmine, lavender

★ **Hives:** Sandalwood

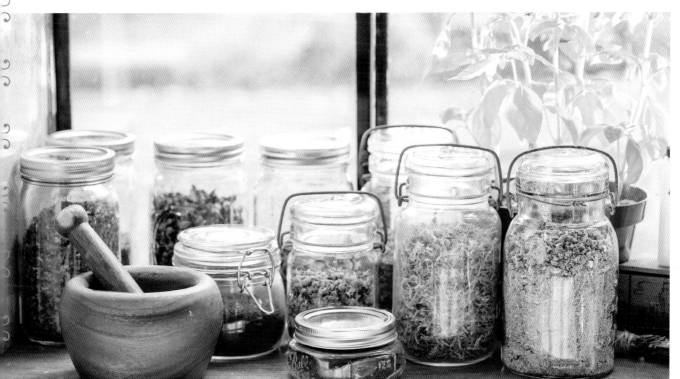

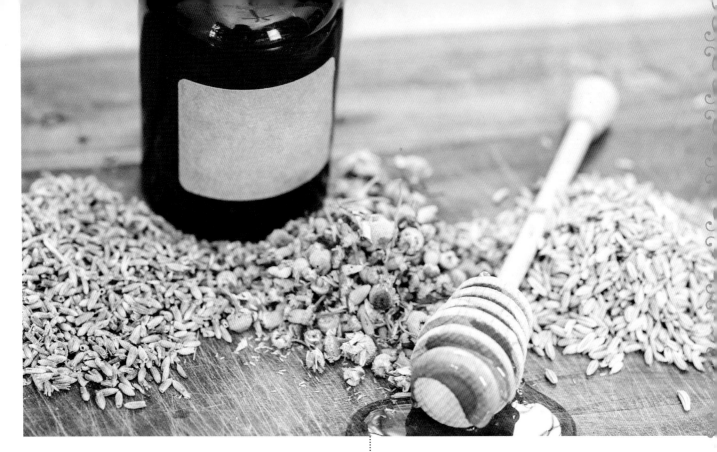

Normal, Mature, or Sensitive Skin Cleanser

This is a gentle cleanser with lavender to soothe and tighten and chamomile to calm. The aloe, glycerin, honey, and jojoba all act as humectants, locking moisture in while also calming irritated or sensitive skin.

INGREDIENTS

FOR HERBAL INFUSION:

1 ounce (28 g) fresh lavender, or
    ½ ounce (14 g) dried lavender
1 ounce (28 g) fresh chamomile, or
    ½ ounce (14 g) dried chamomile
1 quart (1 L) water

⅓ cup (40 g) aloe vera powder
1 cup (235 ml) vegetable glycerin
¼ cup (80 g) honey

15 drops jojoba oil
10 drops rosehip oil

DIRECTIONS

To make the herbal infusion: Follow the directions on page 53.

Combine the infusion with the remaining ingredients in a sterile mixing bowl, and mix well with a hand mixer. Once everything is fully mixed together, pour it into a sterile amber bottle. Store it in a cool place, preferably the refrigerator. After 1 week, discard and start fresh.

To use, place the desired amount onto a facial sponge or washcloth and gently wipe in a circular motion, then rinse with warm water and pat dry. Follow with toner and moisturizer.

Yield: 1 quart (1 L), enough for 1 week's worth of cleanser (depending on amount used)

Oily Skin Cleanser

This is a wonderful cleanser for oily or acne-prone skin; all the herbs work to control oil production, draw out oils, and fight against bacteria. The additional active ingredients aid the skin's healing process and moisturize without clogging pores or leaving the skin greasy.

INGREDIENTS

FOR HERBAL INFUSION:

½ ounce (14 g) dried patchouli seeds

1 ounce (28 g) tea tree leaves

1 ounce (28 g) turmeric

1 ounce (28 g) dried neem leaf

1 ounce (28 g) dried fennel seeds

½ ounce (14 g) dried licorice root (or 2 tablespoons licorice root extract)

2 quarts (2 L) water

⅓ cup (40 g) aloe vera powder

1 cup (235 ml) vegetable glycerin

¼ cup (80 g) honey

15 drops of one of the following (or a mixture): baobab oil, argan oil, camellia oil, grapeseed oil, jojoba oil

5 drops evening primrose oil

DIRECTIONS

TO MAKE THE HERBAL INFUSION: Follow the directions on page 53.

Combine the infusion with the remaining ingredients in a sterile mixing bowl, and mix well with a hand mixer. Once everything is fully mixed together, pour it into a sterile amber bottle. Store it in a cool place, preferably the refrigerator. After 1 week, discard and start fresh.

To use, place the desired amount onto a facial sponge or washcloth and gently wipe in a circular motion, then rinse with warm water and pat dry. Follow with toner and moisturizer.

Yield: 2 quarts (2 L), enough for 1 week's worth of cleanser (depending on amount used)

Dry or Mature Skin Cleanser

This soothing, moisture-enhancing blend of herbs is aided by the natural humectant and skin-soothing effects of aloe, glycerin, and honey.

INGREDIENTS

FOR HERBAL INFUSION:

1 ounce (28 g) dried chamomile
1 ounce (28 g) dried alfalfa
1 ounce (28 g) dried calendula
½ ounce (14 g) dried fennel seeds
1½ quarts (1.5 L) water

⅓ cup (40 g) aloe vera powder
1 cup (235 ml) vegetable glycerin
¼ cup (80 g) honey
15 drops jojoba oil
15 drops apricot kernel oil

DIRECTIONS

TO MAKE THE HERBAL INFUSION: Follow the directions on page 53.

Combine the infusion with the remaining ingredients in a sterile mixing bowl, and mix well with a hand mixer. Once everything is fully mixed together, pour it into a sterile amber bottle. Store it in a cool place, preferably the refrigerator. After 1 week, discard and start fresh.

To use, place the desired amount onto a facial sponge or washcloth and gently wipe in a circular motion, then rinse with warm water and pat dry. Follow with toner and moisturizer.

Yield: 1½ quarts (1.5 L), enough for 1 week's worth of cleanser (depending on amount used)

Basic Makeup Remover

This natural and hydrating solution uses oils as a gentle yet effective way to remove makeup and residue. Such a simple recipe makes it safe enough to act as an eye makeup remover as well.

INGREDIENTS

1 ounce (30 ml) jojoba base oil
½ ounce (15 ml) sweet almond oil
½ ounce (15 ml) vegetable glycerin

DIRECTIONS

Combine all the ingredients and pour the mixture into a sterile, sealable container.

To use, place a small amount on a cotton ball and gently wipe the skin. Follow with your favorite cleanser and toner.

Yield: 2 ounces (60 ml)

These cleansers take their cue from the time-honored cold cream. Cream- or lotion-based cleansers have been used for ages to remove makeup and dirt. They are gentler then harsh-drying surfactant-based cleansers and good for all skin types. These are a little more advanced to make because they require heating, but they are well worth the effort.

To make most creams, lotions, and cream cleansers, heating is required. Without getting too chemistry heavy, we heat the ingredients to make them blend well, and more important, to make oil and water play nice together, for which an emulsifier is often used. As discussed in detail in chapter 3, it's easiest to divide recipes into phases, usually a water phase, an oil phase, and a cool or active ingredient phase (see page 62). All three phases are important; phases A and B kill bacteria and blend the water and oil together, and phase C is necessary to avoid damaging any of the active ingredients.

Normal, Sensitive, Dry, or Mature Skin Cream Cleanser

Rose geranium, which has skin-balancing and hydrating properties, is further enhanced by the addition of rose and aloe vera in this versatile cleanser.

INGREDIENTS

FOR PHASE A:

$\frac{1}{3}$ cup (80 ml) rose herbal infusion (see page 53)

$\frac{1}{3}$ cup (80 ml) rose geranium herbal infusion or rosehip herbal infusion (see page 53)

2 tablespoons (30 ml) aloe vera gel

FOR PHASE B:

2 tablespoons (28 g) vegetable-based emulsifying wax

$\frac{1}{3}$ cup (80 ml) apricot kernel oil

FOR PHASE C:

2 tablespoons (30 ml) vegetable glycerin

1 teaspoon vitamin E oil

10 drops grapefruit seed extract

6 drops palmarosa essential oil

6 drops frankincense essential oil

6 drops patchouli or sandalwood essential oil

1 drop rose geranium essential oil

1 drop jasmine, rose absolute or otto, or ylang ylang essential oil

DIRECTIONS

FOR PHASES A AND B: Follow the directions on page 63 to combine phases A and B at 170°F (77°C).

FOR PHASE C: Once the mixture has cooled to 120°F (49°C) or less, add phase C, continuing to mix.

Once the cleanser has cooled and thickened slightly, pour into a sterilized sealable container, label, and date.

To use, place desired amount onto facial sponge or washcloth and gently wipe in circular motion, rinse with warm water, and pat dry. Follow with toner and moisturizer.

Yield: 1¼ cups (295 ml)

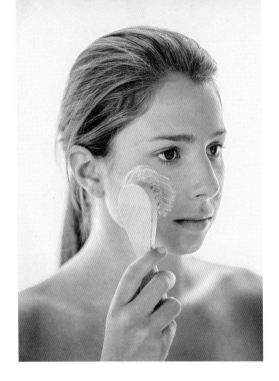

Normal, Dry, or Mature Skin Cream Cleanser

Known for its superior moisturizing abilities, meadowfoam seed oil helps fight against wrinkles and reduces the signs of aging.

INGREDIENTS

FOR PHASE A:

$\frac{1}{4}$ cup (60 ml) meadowfoam seed oil

$1\frac{1}{2}$ teaspoons evening primrose oil

$1\frac{1}{2}$ teaspoons camellia oil

1 tablespoon (15 ml) coconut oil

2 teaspoons rosehip oil

$1\frac{1}{2}$ teaspoons beeswax

FOR PHASE B:

$\frac{1}{4}$ cup (60 ml) aloe vera juice

3 tablespoons (45 ml) distilled water

1 tablespoon (15 ml) vegetable glycerin

$\frac{1}{4}$ teaspoon borax

FOR PHASE C:

15 drops lavender essential oil

5 drops rose absolute or rose otto oil

DIRECTIONS

FOR PHASES A AND B: Follow the directions on page 63 to combine phases A and B at 170°F (77°C).

FOR PHASE C: Once the mixture has cooled to 120°F (49°C) or less, add phase C, continuing to mix.

Once the cleanser has cooled and thickened slightly, pour into a sterilized sealable container, label, and date.

To use, place desired amount onto facial sponge or washcloth and gently wipe in circular motion, rinse with warm water, and pat dry. Follow with a toner and moisturizer.

Yield: 1 cup (235 ml)

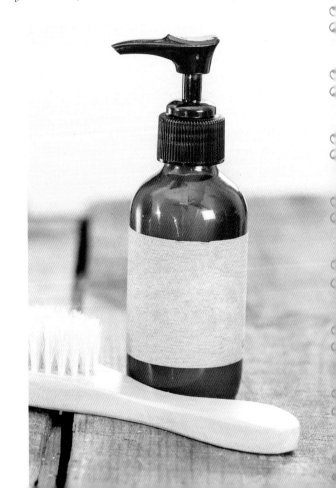

Sensitive or Dry Skin Cream Cleanser

A favorite, this cleanser leaves the skin moisturized and refreshed. This cleanser is great for the winter months when the skin is at its driest.

INGREDIENTS

1¹⁄₂ teaspoons sunflower oil
1¹⁄₂ teaspoons olive oil
1¹⁄₂ teaspoons jojoba oil
1 tablespoon cocoa butter
1¹⁄₂ teaspoons soy wax or beeswax
1¹⁄₂ teaspoons vegetable glycerin
2 drops chamomile essential oil
2 drops lavender essential oil

DIRECTIONS

Melt the sunflower oil, olive oil, jojoba oil, cocoa butter, and wax together in a double boiler. Once fully melted, remove from the heat and slowly add the glycerin while stirring. The mixture will start to thicken. Add the essential oils and transfer to a sterile container to cool.

To use, massage a small amount into the skin in a circular motion with your fingertips. Rinse with warm water, pat dry, and follow with toner and moisturizer.

Yield: ¼ cup (60 ml)

Oily or Combination Skin Cream Cleanser

The antimicrobial effects of neem oil combined with an essential oil blend to fight oils and acne make this cleanser great for oily and combination skin types.

INGREDIENTS

FOR PHASE A:
¹⁄₂ cup (120 ml) distilled water
¹⁄₄ cup (54 g) borax

FOR PHASE B:
¹⁄₄ cup (60 ml) hazelnut oil
1 teaspoon neem oil
1 tablespoon (15 ml) coconut oil
1 teaspoon beeswax

FOR PHASE C:
5 drops rosemary essential oil
5 drops sage oil
5 drops goldenseal leaf oil

DIRECTIONS

FOR PHASES A AND B: Follow the directions on page 63 to combine phases A and B at 170°F (77°C).

FOR PHASE C: Once the mixture has cooled to 120°F (49°C) or less, add phase C, continuing to mix.

Once the cleanser has cooled and thickened slightly, pour into a sterilized sealable container, label, and date.

To use, massage a small amount into the skin in a circular motion with your fingertips. Rinse with warm water, pat dry, and follow with toner and moisturizer.

Yield: 1 cup (235 ml)

Oily or Combination Skin Cream Cleanser

This gentle cleanser combines carrier oils targeted to help heal and tone oily or combination skin. It unclogs pores and deep cleans.

INGREDIENTS

FOR PHASE A:

½ cup (120 ml) witch hazel
2 tablespoons (30 ml) aloe vera gel

FOR PHASE B:

2 tablespoons (28 g) emulsifying wax
2 tablespoons (30 ml) grapeseed oil
2 tablespoons (30 ml) hazelnut oil
1 tablespoon (15 ml) apricot kernel oil
1 teaspoon neem oil
1 teaspoon vitamin E oil

FOR PHASE C:

10 drops fennel essential oil
5 drops tea tree essential oil
5 drops peppermint essential oil
5 drops thyme essential oil

DIRECTIONS

FOR PHASES A AND B: Follow the directions on page 63 to combine phases A and B at 170°F (77°C).

FOR PHASE C: Once the mixture has cooled to 120°F (49°C) or less, add phase C, continuing to mix.

Once the cleanser has cooled and thickened slightly, pour into a sterilized sealable container, label, and date.

To use, massage a small amount into the skin in a circular motion with your fingertips. Rinse with warm water, pat dry, and follow with toner and moisturizer.

Yield: 1 cup (235 ml)

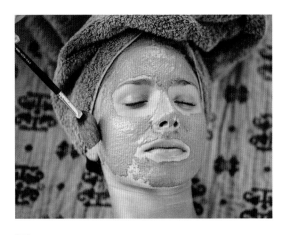

POWDERED CLEANSERS

Powdered cleansers are a great alternative to regular cleansers. Because they are powdered, they have a longer shelf life. They are full of skin-beautifying benefits, and they can also double as your weekly mask, saving you money.

To apply a powdered cleanser or mask, simply spoon some into the palm of your hand and apply a wetting agent (see below) to create a paste. Apply to your face and neck, avoiding the eye area. Leave on for 2 to 5 minutes, and then rinse off.

There are many options when it comes to wetting agents, from plain old water to milk, almond milk, or honey. Or get creative and combine fruit juices and/or an herbal infusion of your choice. See chapter 8 for some seasonal wetting agent ideas. My personal favorite is honey. Alternatively, you can combine a powdered cleanser with a cream cleanser as your wetting agent.

Powdered cleansers, if kept dry and sealed, have a very long shelf life. The recipes below yield 6 to 10 ounces (168 to 280 g), which is not all needed for a single treatment. These powders can be stored for later use as long as the wetting agent isn't added.

Powdered Cleanser for Mature or Dry Skin

This combination of moisture-replenishing clays reduces the appearance of wrinkles by tightening the skin, fighting the signs of aging.

INGREDIENTS

½ cup (60 g) kaolin clay
⅓ cup (40 g) oat flour or rice flour
⅓ cup (40 g) rosehip powder
¼ cup (30 g) rhassoul clay
1 tablespoon (14 g) powdered lavender
1 tablespoon (14 g) powdered rose petals

DIRECTIONS

Combine all the ingredients in a bowl until well blended, and then transfer to a clean, moisture-free container.

To use, spoon some cleanser into the palm of your hand and apply a wetting agent (see page 80) to create a paste. Apply to your face and neck, avoiding the eye area. Leave on for 2 to 5 minutes, and then rinse off.

Yield: 1½ cups (180 g)

Gentle Powdered Cleanser

This gentle cleanser with the skin-calming properties of chamomile cleanses the skin without irritating. This cleanser is great for all skin types, even sensitive skin. It leaves the skin refreshed, moisturized, and bright.

INGREDIENTS

½ cup (40 g) rolled oats
½ cup (60 g) powdered goat's milk (if unavailable just double the rolled oats)
¼ cup (20 g) powdered chamomile or lavender (if unavailable add 1 table-spoon dried chamomile)
1½ cups (355 ml) soy milk or almond milk
1 tablespoon (20 g) honey

DIRECTIONS

Blend all the ingredients in a blender until creamy. This recipe can be stored in a sealed sterile container in the refrigerator for up to a week. Alternatively, mix the dry ingredients and store in a sealed container, adding the soy milk and honey when ready to use.

To use, apply the cleanser to the face with a gentle circular motion. Rinse well with warm water.

Yield: 2¾ cups (500 g)

Powdered Cleanser for Oily Skin

Deep cleaning and pore refining, this is a great cleanser for problem skin.

INGREDIENTS

$1/2$ cup (60 g) kaolin clay
$1/4$ cup (30 g) neem powder
$1/4$ cup (30 g) fennel powder
$1/4$ cup (30 g) bentonite clay

DIRECTIONS

Combine all the ingredients in a bowl until well blended and then transfer to a clean, moisture-free container.

To use, apply the cleanser to the face with a gentle circular motion. Rinse well with warm water.

Yield: 1 1/4 cups (150 g)

FACIAL SCRUBS

Facial scrubs are similar to powdered cleansers in that they act as an exfoliant, but they are rinsed off immediately, unlike masks, which stay on the skin for several minutes. Exfoliating the skin is essential: it helps slough off dead skin cells and gets deep into pores to remove dirt and oil, revealing a healthy glow. Scrubs also allow your lotion to work better.

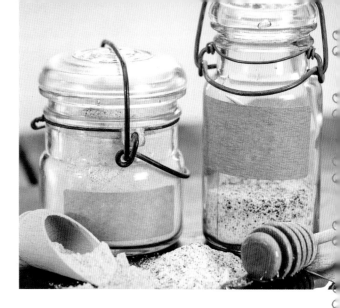

Gentle Facial Exfoliant

This cleanser is great for all skin types, especially sensitive skin, and leaves the skin refreshed, moisturized, and bright.

INGREDIENTS

1 cup (120 g) powdered cow or goat's milk
$1/2$ cup (40 g) rolled oats
$1/4$ cup (35 g) cornmeal
$1/4$ cup (30 g) powdered chamomile or lavender (if unavailable add 1 tablespoon dried chamomile finely ground with a mortar and pestle)
1 tablespoon (20 g) honey (to be used as wetting agent; amount can be adjusted as needed)

DIRECTIONS

Combine the dry ingredients and mix well. This mixture can be stored in a dry container for several applications; add the wetting agent only at the time of use.

To use, apply the cleanser to the face in a gentle circular motion. Rinse well with warm water.

Yield: 2 cups (245 g)

Almond Scrub for All Skin Types

Rich in phytochemicals, almonds help treat a variety of skin aliments with their antioxidant and astringent properties. Sunflower seeds are full of vitamin E, decelerating the aging of skin cells and diminishing the appearance of scars.

INGREDIENTS

2 tablespoons (14 g) finely ground almonds
1 tablespoon (7 g) ground sunflower seeds
1 tablespoon (5 g) oatmeal
1 tablespoon (7 g) wheat germ
1 tablespoon (8 g) chamomile powder
Sweet almond oil, water, honey, or milk (to be used as wetting agent, amount can be adjusted as needed)

DIRECTIONS

Combine all the ingredients in a blender until creamy. Alternatively, you can double the recipe, combine only the dry ingredients, and store in dry, sealed container for several applications, add wetting agents only at the time of use.

To use, apply to the face in a gentle circular motion. Rinse well with warm water.

Yield: 3 ounces (42 g)

Exfoliator for Oily or Combination Skin

This creamy exfoliating mask uses almonds, orange peel, and peppermint to draw out oils and fight acne. This mixture will exfoliate the skin without overdrying or irritating it.

INGREDIENTS

$\frac{1}{2}$ cup (60 g) kaolin clay
$\frac{1}{4}$ cup (30 g) finely ground almonds
$\frac{1}{2}$ cup (60 g) powdered goat's milk
2 tablespoons (15 g) cornmeal
2 teaspoons powdered orange peel
2 teaspoons dried peppermint leaves
Honey, water, or jojoba oil (to be used as wetting agent, amount can be adjusted as needed)

DIRECTIONS

Combine the dry ingredients, mix well, and store in a dry sealed container until ready to use. Add the wetting agent only at the time of use.

To use, apply to the face in a gentle circular motion. Rinse well with warm water.

Yield: 1 $\frac{1}{2}$ cups (180 g)

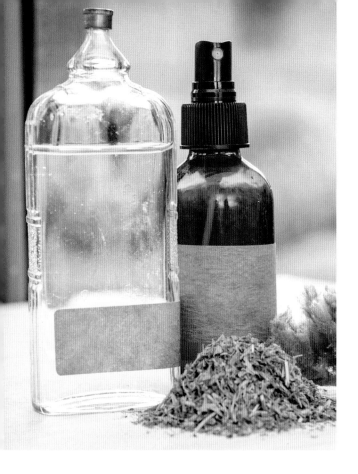

Toners and Astringents

Toners contain moisturizers, oils, and extracts that help soothe your skin. Astringents tighten the skin and pores and remove oil. Both toners and astringents assist in reducing the appearance of large pores and exfoliate the skin while removing any residual buildup your cleanser may have left behind.

Rose Water Toner

Rose water retains moisture, fighting the signs of aging and balancing the skin. This toner is soothing and nourishing for all skin types, especially dry, mature, and sensitive types.

INGREDIENTS

½ cup (120 ml) distilled water
½ cup (120 ml) rose water (can also use rose or rosehip infusion, see page 53)
¼ cup (60 ml) witch hazel
1 tablespoon (14 g) aloe vera gel or aloe vera powder

DIRECTIONS

Mix all the ingredients together. Pour the mixture into a sterile container, label it, and date it.

To use, moisten a cotton facial pad with toner. Wipe gently in small circles, focusing on the forehead, nose, and chin. Be careful to avoid the delicate eye area. Follow with moisturizer.

Yield: 1¼ cups (300 ml)

Problem Skin Toner

The antiseptic and antibacterial properties of tea tree oil, thyme, and black willow bark fight acne-causing bacteria and oils, revealing toned, balanced skin.

INGREDIENTS

½ cup (120 ml) distilled water
¼ cup (60 ml) witch hazel
¾ teaspoon aloe vera gel
10 drops tea tree essential oil
5 drops black willow bark essential oil
5 drops thyme essential oil

DIRECTIONS

Mix all the ingredients together. Pour the mixture into a sterile container, label it, and date it.

To use, moisten a cotton facial pad with toner. Wipe gently in small circles, focusing on the forehead, nose, and chin. Be careful to avoid the delicate eye area. Follow with a moisturizer.

Yield: ¾ cup (180 ml)

Green Tea Toner

This toner is great for all skin types. Packed full of antioxidants, green tea works wonders on mature, dry skin, yet its soothing properties are great on aggravated skin as well.

INGREDIENTS

1 cup (235 ml) distilled water
2 tablespoons (15 g) green tea leaves
¼ cup (60 ml) witch hazel
1 teaspoon vegetable glycerin

DIRECTIONS

Make an herbal infusion using the distilled water and tea leaves (see page 53). Add the witch hazel and glycerin to the infusion and mix well. Pour the mixture into a sterile container, label it, and date it.

To use, moisten a cotton facial pad with toner. Wipe gently in small circles, focusing on the forehead, nose, and chin. Be careful to avoid the delicate eye area. Follow with a moisturizer.

Yield: 1¼ cups (300 ml)

Acne Toner

Yarrow and calendula soothe and heal damaged skin and help prevent scars, while the antibacterial effects of patchouli and tea tree fight acne-causing bacteria. This toner is soothing and refreshing for oily, problematic skin.

INGREDIENTS

```
2 cups (470 ml) distilled water
1 tablespoon dried yarrow
1 tablespoon dried calendula leaves
1 teaspoon freshly squeezed lemon juice
1 tablespoon (20 g) honey
¼ cup (60 ml) witch hazel
4 drops patchouli essential oil
3 drops tea tree essential oil
```

DIRECTIONS

Make an herbal infusion using the distilled water, yarrow, and calendula (see page 53). Add the lemon juice, honey, witch hazel, and essential oils to the infusion. Pour into a sterile container, label it, and date it.

To use, moisten a cotton facial pad with toner. Wipe gently in small circles, focusing on the forehead, nose, and chin. Be careful to avoid the delicate eye area. Follow with a moisturizer.

Yield: 2¼ cups (530 ml)

Healing Facial Tonic

If you're surprised to see marshmallow root as a healing element, consider this: it's actually where roasting marshmallows around the campfire started. Parents used to roast the root in the fire (their stove at the time) for their children to ease sore throats and coughs.

INGREDIENTS

```
2 cups (470 ml) distilled water
1 teaspoon chopped comfrey root
1 teaspoon chopped marshmallow root
1 teaspoon dried chamomile
1 teaspoon dried calendula
2 tablespoons (30 ml) witch hazel
1 teaspoon vegetable glycerin
5 drops lavender essential oil
5 drops juniper essential oil
```

DIRECTIONS

Make a decoction using the distilled water and herbs (see page 55). Add the witch hazel, glycerin, and essential oils to the decoction. Pour into a sterile container, label it, and date it.

To use, moisten a cotton facial pad with toner. Wipe gently in small circles, focusing on the forehead, nose, and chin. Be careful to avoid the delicate eye area. Follow with a moisturizer.

Yield: 2 cups (470 ml)

Sensitive Skin Toner

Rose petals and chamomile soothe and nourish the skin, while orange blossoms calm and brighten. This toner is great for dry and sensitive skin types.

INSTRUCTIONS

3 cups (705 ml) distilled water

2 tablespoons dried rose petals

2 tablespoons dried chamomile

3 tablespoons dried orange blossom flower

1/4 cup (60 ml) witch hazel

5 drops jasmine essential oil

5 drops neroli essential oil

DIRECTIONS

Make an herbal infusion using the distilled water and herbs (see page 53). Add the witch hazel and essential oils to the infusion and mix well. Pour into a sterile container, label it, and date it.

To use, moisten a cotton facial pad with toner. Wipe gently in small circles, focusing on the forehead, nose, and chin. Be careful to avoid the delicate eye area. Follow with a moisturizer.

Yield: 3 1/4 cups (765 ml)

CREAMS AND LOTIONS

An essential part of your skin care regimen, moisturizer should be applied after cleansing twice a day. Here you'll find recipes tailored to specific skin needs. And for those of you who prefer to customize your own formula, there are some sample base recipes to start from.

Cream for Mature, Dry, and Sensitive Skin

Chamomile soothes while lavender and elderflower moisturize.

INGREDIENTS

FOR PHASE A:

3 cups (705 ml) distilled water

3 tablespoons dried elderflowers

2 tablespoons dried chamomile

2 tablespoons dried lavender

1 tablespoon comfrey

1/2 teaspoon borax

FOR PHASE B:

2 tablespoons (28 g) emulsifying wax

1 teaspoon beeswax

2 1/2 tablespoons (37 ml) sweet almond oil

2 teaspoons coconut oil

FOR PHASE C:

10 drops frankincense essential oil

5 drops palmarosa essential oil

DIRECTIONS

FOR PHASE A: Make an herbal infusion with the distilled water and herbs (see page 53). Heat the infusion in a double boiler and add the borax.

FOR PHASE B: In a separate double boiler heat the phase B ingredients. Follow the directions on page 63 to combine phases A and B at 170°F (77°C). Stir frequently as it cools.

FOR PHASE C: Once the mixture has cooled to 120°F (49°C) or less, mix in phase C.

Once the mixture has cooled, pour into a sterilized sealable container, label, and date.

To use, after cleansing and toning, apply lotion in a circular motion. Be careful around the eyes.

Yield: 3 cups (705 ml)

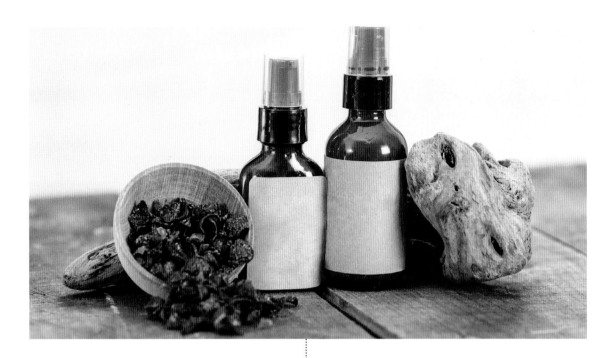

Lotion for Oily or Combination Skin

Calendula, a natural antimicrobial, helps regulate oily skin while healing inflammation.

INGREDIENTS

FOR PHASE A:

1 tablespoon (15 ml) vegetable glycerin

$\frac{1}{3}$ cup (80 ml) distilled water

FOR PHASE B:

2 tablespoons (28 g) emulsifying wax

$\frac{1}{4}$ cup (60 ml) jojoba oil

$\frac{1}{4}$ cup (60 ml) apricot kernel oil

FOR PHASE C:

1 teaspoon vitamin E oil

10 drops grapefruit seed extract

4 drops calendula essential oil

3 drops patchouli essential oil

2 drops rose geranium essential oil

2 drops tea tree essential oil

DIRECTIONS

For phases A and B: Follow the directions on page 63 to combine phases A and B at 170°F (77°C).

FOR PHASE C: Once the mixture has cooled to 120°F (49°C) or less, add phase C, and stir constantly until cool. Store in a sterile container, label it, and date it.

To use, after cleansing and toning, apply lotion in a circular motion. Be careful around the delicate eye area.

Yield: 1 cup (235 ml)

Basic Lotion Base

The next two recipes are great base lotions that then allow you to customize the essentials oils to your needs or preferences. The oils used are beneficial for all skin types, but as you experiment more, these too can be substituted to your liking.

INGREDIENTS

FOR PHASE A:
1¼ cups (295 ml) distilled water

FOR PHASE B:
¼ cup (60 ml) sweet almond oil
¼ cup (60 ml) evening primrose oil
2 tablespoons (30 ml) meadowfoam seed oil
3 tablespoons (42 g) emulsifying wax

FOR PHASE C:
15 drops essential oil of your choice

DIRECTIONS

FOR PHASES A AND B: Follow the directions on page 63 to combine phases A and B at 170°F (77°C).

FOR PHASE C: Once the mixture has cooled to 120°F (49°C) or less, add phase C, and stir constantly until cool. Store in a sterile container, label it, and date it.

To use, after cleansing and toning, apply lotion in a circular motion. Be careful around the delicate eye area.

Yield: 2 cups (470 ml)

Basic Cream Base

Here is another great basic cream that can be made with your choice of infusion or decoction.

INGREDIENTS

FOR PHASE A:
½ cup (120 ml) herbal infusion (page 53) or decoction (page 55) best suited for your skin (see page 70)

FOR PHASE B:
1 tablespoon (14 g) beeswax
2 teaspoons emulsifying wax
2 tablespoons (30 ml) coconut oil
2 teaspoons avocado oil

FOR PHASE C:
20 drops essential oils of your choice

DIRECTIONS

FOR PHASES A AND B: Follow the directions on page 63 to combine phases A and B at 170°F (77°C).

FOR PHASE C: Once the mixture has cooled to 120°F (49°C) or less, add phase C, and stir constantly until cool. Store in a sterile container, label it, and date it.

To use, after cleansing and toning, apply lotion in a circular motion. Be careful around the delicate eye area.

Yield: ¾ cup (180 ml)

TREATMENT OILS AND GENTLE CLEANSERS

These recipes can be used either as gentle cleansers or as treatment oils that can be left on the skin for added moisture and skin-healing benefits. Oils are great to use as substitutes for traditional cleansers, especially on extremely dry or irritated skin. They remove dirt without stripping the skin's natural oils.

Light Moisturizing Oil or Cleanser

This is a great moisturizing oil or cleanser for sensitive skin types.

INGREDIENTS

½ cup (120 ml) distilled water (omit if used as a treatment oil)
2 teaspoons vegetable glycerin (substitute ¼ cup [60 ml] jojoba or borage oil if this will be used as a treatment oil)
5 drops chamomile essential oil
2 drops lavender essential oil

DIRECTIONS

Blend all the ingredients well and store in a sterile container.

To use as a treatment oil, apply a few drops to your fingertips and massage onto skin; do not rinse. To use as a cleanser, apply about 1 tablespoon (15 ml) of the mixture to your face in a circular motion. Rinse and pat dry, then follow with toner and moisturizer.

Yield: ½ cup (120 ml) cleanser or ¼ cup (60 ml) treatment oil

Acne Skin Treatment Oil or Cleanser

This blend of essential oils helps cleanse bacteria and refreshes the skin without overdrying or irritating it. It's great for those with combination skin.

INGREDIENTS

½ cup (120 ml) distilled water (substitute ¼ cup [60 ml] jojoba or grapeseed oil if used as a treatment oil)
5 drops rosemary essential oil
5 drops thyme essential oil
2 drops lemon essential oil
6 drops German chamomile essential oil
4 drops sage essential oil
¼ cup (60 ml) hazelnut oil

DIRECTIONS

Blend all the ingredients well and store in a sterile container.

To use as a treatment oil, apply a few drops to the fingertips and massage onto skin; do not rinse. To use as a cleanser, apply 1 tablespoon (15 ml) of the mixture to the face in a circular motion. Rinse and pat dry, then follow with a toner and moisturizer of your choice.

Yield: ¾ cup (180 ml) cleanser or ½ cup (120 ml) treatment oil

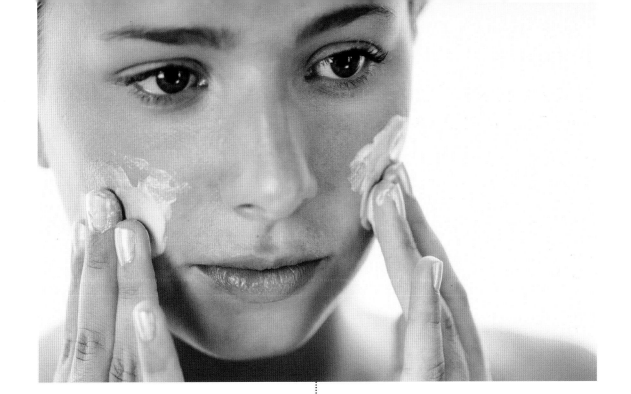

Mature Skin Treatment Oil or Cleanser

Carrot seed oil is a favorite for fighting the signs of aging; combined with the nourishing properties of rosehip and argan, this is a powerful moisturizing treatment when used either as a cleanser or as a treatment oil.

INGREDIENTS

½ cup (120 ml) distilled water (omit if used as a treatment oil)

7 drops carrot seed essential oil

7 drops helichrysum essential oil

6 drops calendula essential oil

1 tablespoon (15 ml) rosehip seed oil

1 teaspoon meadowfoam seed oil

2 teaspoons argan oil

DIRECTIONS

Blend all the ingredients well and store in a sterile container.

To use as a treatment oil, apply a few drops to the fingertips and massage onto skin; do not rinse. To use as a cleanser, apply 1 tablespoon (15 ml) of the mixture to the face in a circular motion. Rinse and pat dry, then follow with a toner and moisturizer of your choice.

Yield: ½ cup (120 ml) cleanser or 2 tablespoons (30 ml) treatment oil

Facial Treatments and Serums

Facial treatments are geared to solving a specific aliment; most often they are spot treatments or eye treatments. Facial serums are often used in conjunction with your every-day moisturizer or in times of need.

Soothing Facial Serum

This serum features the calming and healing effects of calendula and comfrey essential oils.

INGREDIENTS

1 tablespoon (15 ml) rosehip oil
1 tablespoon (15 ml) papaya seed oil
2 tablespoons (30 ml) meadowfoam seed oil
4 drops calendula essential oil
2 drops comfrey essential oil

DIRECTIONS

Blend all the ingredients well and store in a sterile container. When properly stored, this oil will keep for 3 to 6 months.

To use, after cleansing and toning, apply a few drops to clean fingertips and gently rub onto skin. Can be followed with a moisturizer if needed.

Yield: ¼ cup (60 ml)

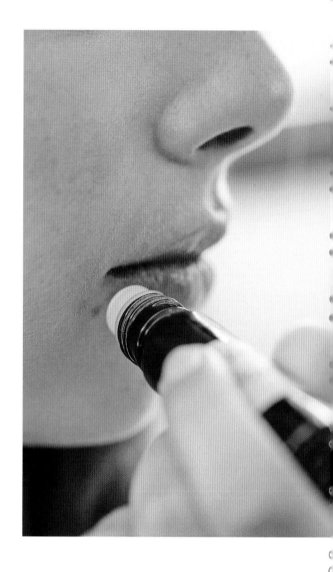

Acne Spot Treatment

Acne isn't this treatment's only use; it also works well as an antimicrobial for minor scrapes and irritations.

INGREDIENTS

1 tablespoon (20 g) organic honey

1 teaspoon neem oil

5 drops tea tree essential oil

5 drops goldenseal leaf essential oil

DIRECTIONS

Blend all the ingredients well and store in a sterile container, preferably in the refrigerator.

To use, dab a small amount on the affected area.

Yield: 1½ tablespoons (23 ml)

Blackhead Spot Treatment

This simple recipe is a quick fix for those annoying blackheads. Parsley helps extract and prevent blackheads, especially with continued use.

INGREDIENTS

2 tablespoons (3 g) dried parsley flakes

3 tablespoons (45 ml) witch hazel

DIRECTIONS

With a mortar and pestle, mash together the parsley flakes and witch hazel. Store in sterile container in the refrigerator.

To use, apply to the affected area and let sit for 5 to 10 minutes. It can be applied as often as needed or until the condition improves.

Yield: ¼ cup (60 ml)

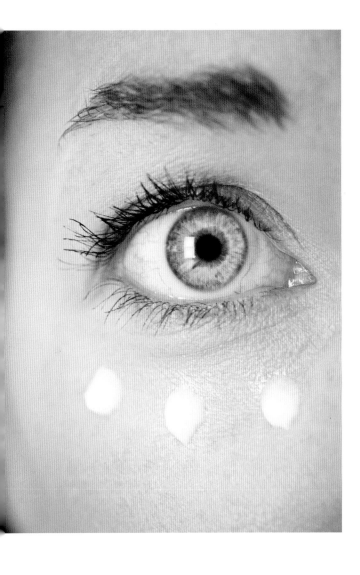

Eye Treatments

A common complaint among us all is the under-eye area. This delicate skin is prone to puffiness and is the first to show signs of aging. The following recipes will help alleviate those problems.

Cucumber Eye Gel

This hydrating eye gel soothes and calms tired eyes. Cucumber juice and aloe vera act like an instant drink of water for your skin, hydrating thirsty cells.

INGREDIENTS

1 tablespoon (14 g) aloe vera gel
1 teaspoon fresh cucumber juice,
  strained (best it you have a juicer)
¼ teaspoon cornstarch
1 tablespoon (15 ml) witch hazel

DIRECTIONS

In a double boiler, combine the aloe, cucumber juice, and cornstarch and warm carefully; be careful not to overheat or bring to a boil. Remove and transfer to a bowl, and mix in the witch hazel. Allow to cool completely before transferring the mixture to a sterile container. This gel will last a week if properly stored; it's best to store in the refrigerator, and doing so also makes it a refreshing eye treatment.

To use, apply under the eye in an upward, dotting motion, being careful not to pull on the skin.

Yield: 2 tablespoons (30 ml)

Chamomile Eye Salve

The delicate skin around the eyes is the first to show signs of aging and stress. Chamomile reduces dark circles and puffiness with its anti-inflammatory properties.

INGREDIENTS

5 tablespoons (70 g) shea butter

1 tablespoon (14 g) beeswax

2 tablespoons (30 ml) sweet almond oil

5 drops chamomile essential oil

2 drops palmarosa essential oil

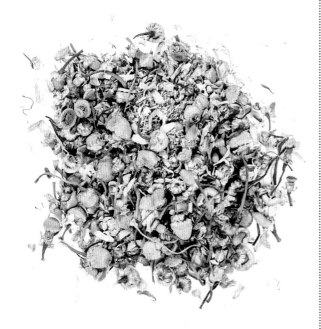

DIRECTIONS

Melt the shea butter, beeswax, and almond oil in a double boiler, stirring gently, then remove from the heat. Let cool to at least 120°F (49°C), and add the essential oils before it begins to solidify. Pour into a sterile container and let cool until solid.

To use, apply under the eye in an upward, dotting motion, being careful not to pull on the skin.

Yield: ½ cup (115 g)

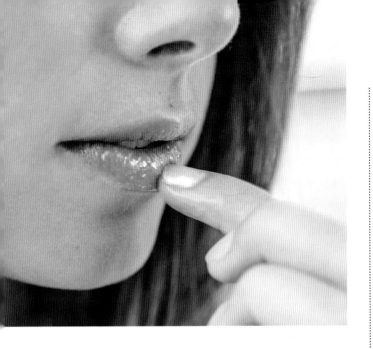

LIP TREATMENTS

Lip balms and glosses are easy to make and fun to experiment with. You can customize them to your needs, and they make great gifts for friends and family.

Lip-Plumping Moisture Gloss

A great moisturizing balm, this recipe uses anise and cinnamon essential oils to create a gentle, natural plumping effect. To add color to the gloss, you can stir in beet juice or beet powder.

INGREDIENTS

2 teaspoons beeswax
2 teaspoons coconut oil
1/4 teaspoon vitamin E oil
2 tablespoons (30 ml) sweet almond oil
2 or 3 drops cinnamon essential oil
2 drops anise essential oil

DIRECTIONS

Place the beeswax, coconut oil, vitamin E oil, and almond oil in a double boiler over medium heat. Stir until melted and remove from the heat. Slowly stir in the essential oils. Slowly pour into a sealable, sterile container. Let cool and solidify before using.

To use, apply to the lips as needed.

Yield: 3 tablespoons (45 ml)

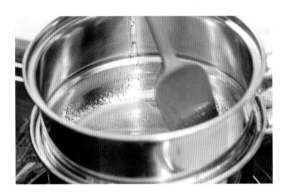

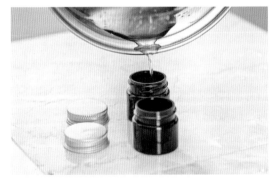

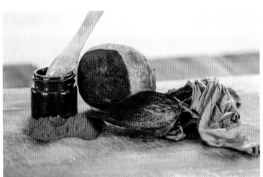

Exfoliating Lip Treatment

This is a great and easy treatment for exfoliating dry, chapped lips.

INGREDIENTS

1½ tablespoons (23 ml) apricot
  kernel oil
2 teaspoons organic honey
1 tablespoon (15 g) coarse brown
  sugar

DIRECTIONS

In a clean bowl, mix together all the ingredients. Pour into a sealable, sterile container.

To use, gently rub the mixture onto your lips with a clean fingertip, then rinse.

Yield: 3 tablespoons (45 ml)

Vanilla Lip Balm

This recipe makes a simple and tasty lip balm.

INGREDIENTS

1 teaspoon organic honey
2 tablespoons (30 ml) sweet almond oil
2 teaspoons beeswax
½ teaspoon candelilla wax
5 drops vanilla extract

DIRECTIONS

In a clean bowl, mix together all the ingredients. Pour into a sealable, sterile container.

To use, gently rub the mixture onto your lips with a clean fingertip.

Yield: 3 tablespoons (45 ml)

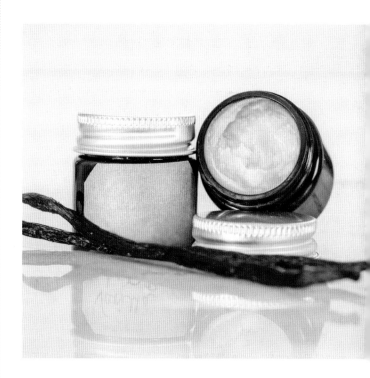

NATURAL SUN PROTECTION

Although the sun is a valuable source of vitamin D, protecting yourself from its damaging effects is very important for healthy, youthful skin. You'll find there are tons of chemicals in most of the sunscreens on the market today. However, there are several natural alternatives, such as titanium dioxide and zinc oxide, that create a reflective barrier to the sun. (Most mineral makeups are made from these.) Here are some other natural alternatives, which can be used alone or in combination to increase the spf:

Avocado oil: Rich in antioxidants and vitamins A and E, this nourishing oil won't clog pores and penetrates the skin easily. It has an SPF of 8.

* *

Buriti fruit oil: Rich in essential fatty acids and carotenoids, including beta-carotene, buriti fruit oil protects the skin from free radical damage and heals the effects of sun damage. It also processes a natural SPF factor.

* *

Carrot seed oil: This oil, with its antioxidant-rich levels of vitamin A, has an SPF of 15 to 30. Be sure to dilute it in a carrier oil (see page 38).

* *

Grapeseed oil: Packed full powerful antioxidants, grapeseed oil promotes repair from sun damage. It has an SPF of 4.

Jojoba oil: This carrier oil is close to that of our own natural sebum, so it is not only great for healing dry, irritated skin, but it also has an SPF of around 4.

* *

Neem oil: Not only does this oil work wonders on damaged skin, clearing blemishes and healing wounds, but it also has a natural SPF of about 2.

* *

Red raspberry seed oil: With high levels of essential fatty acids and the antioxidant vitamin E, this oil boasts a natural SPF of 30 to 50.

* *

Sesame oil: Rich in vitamin E, sesame oil is great for very dry skin, and it has an SPF of 4.

* *

Shea butter: Absorbing rapidly into the skin, shea butter contains cinnamic acid, which provides ultraviolet ray protection. It's also great to use after sun exposure because it is rich in antioxidants and vitamins A and E, and it possesses superior skin-hydrating abilities. It has a natural SPF of about 8.

Red Raspberry Seed Oil Natural Sunscreen Balm

This balm bar works great as a natural SPF. The beeswax in the recipe adds a nice water-proof property and the oils all act to protect the skin as well as aid in healing damaged skin.

INGREDIENTS

2 tablespoons (30 ml) red raspberry seed oil

1 tablespoon (15 ml) buriti fruit oil

1 tablespoon (15 ml) avocado oil (or any other of the carrier oils from page 98)

2 ounces (54 g) beeswax

2 ounces (54 g) shea butter

2 teaspoons vitamin E oil

1½ tablespoons (11 g) zinc oxide or titanium oxide

20 drops carrot seed oil

DIRECTIONS

In a double boiler, melt the red raspberry seed oil, buriti fruit oil, avocado oil, beeswax, shea butter, and vitamin E oil. Remove from the heat and allow to cool for a bit before adding the zinc oxide and carrot seed oil. You can put this balm in a round glass container, a tin, or a large push-up lip balm or deodorant container.

To use, apply as needed.

Yield: 7 ounces (196 g)

Sun Relief Treatments

There are numerous essentials oils that can help soothe the skin after sun damage. Essential oils that can be added to sun relief recipes are lavender, sandalwood, chamomile, and rose otto or absolute.

Chamomile Sun Relief Infusion

Chamomile is known for its soothing effects on the body both internally and externally. This infusion works amazingly well to soothe and take the sting out of sunburn. It's great to keep on hand in the refrigerator as a cooling skin treatment after a (too long) day in the sun.

INGREDIENTS

1 to 2 tablespoons (2 to 4 g) dried chamomile
1 cup (235 ml) water
2 tablespoons (30 ml) apple cider vinegar

DIRECTIONS

Make an infusion with the chamomile and water following the directions on page 53. Add the apple cider vinegar. Pour the mixture into a sterile spray bottle and place it in the refrigerator to cool.

To use, spray on the affected area (do not rub on the skin) and let dry. Reapply as needed.

Yield: 1 cup (235 ml)

→ KITCHEN RESCUES ←

Here are some quick body care rescues that you'll find in your kitchen.

* **Apple cider vinegar:** Add 1 to 2 cups (235 to 470 ml) to bathwater and soak to help relieve sunburn or aggravated skin conditions.

* **Black pekoe tea:** Apply directly to sunburn.

* **Dried chamomile:** Make an infusion (see page 53) and let it cool in the fridge. Once chilled, spray directly onto the burned area.

* **Lemon juice:** Removes sunless tanner. Simply rub lemon slices or a cotton ball dampened with lemon juice on the area of concern.

* **Raw potato:** Apply to burns and scrapes, and to take the itch out of bug bites.

* **Yogurt:** Apply to a sunburn to relieve pain.

Lavender Aloe Spray

This recipe is a favorite of mine! I always have this on hand during the summer months; not only is it super refreshing and hydrating to the skin, but its soothing effects also feel great on sunburned skin.

INGREDIENTS

1 cup (235 ml) aloe vera gel (oil extract or powder can also be used)
½ cup (120 ml) witch hazel
½ cup (120 ml) distilled water
15 drops lavender essential oil

DIRECTIONS

Pour all the ingredients into a sterile spray bottle, seal, and shake. Place in the refrigerator to cool.

To use, spray on the affected area (do not rub on the skin) and let dry. Reapply as needed.

Yield: 2 cups (470 ml)

Sun Relief Milk

Very soothing to the skin, this combination relieves the pain of sunburn while helping heal the skin with the hydrating effects of aloe and the anti-inflammatory properties of cucumber.

INGREDIENTS

½ cup (120 ml) aloe vera juice
½ cup (120 ml) cucumber juice
1 cup (235 ml) buttermilk
10 drops lavender essential oil

DIRECTIONS

Combine all the ingredients in a bowl, and soak some cheesecloth or muslin strips in the mixture.

To use, apply the strips to the sunburned area and let sit. Alternatively, you can pour the mixture into a bath and use as a soak.

Yield: 2 cups (470 ml)

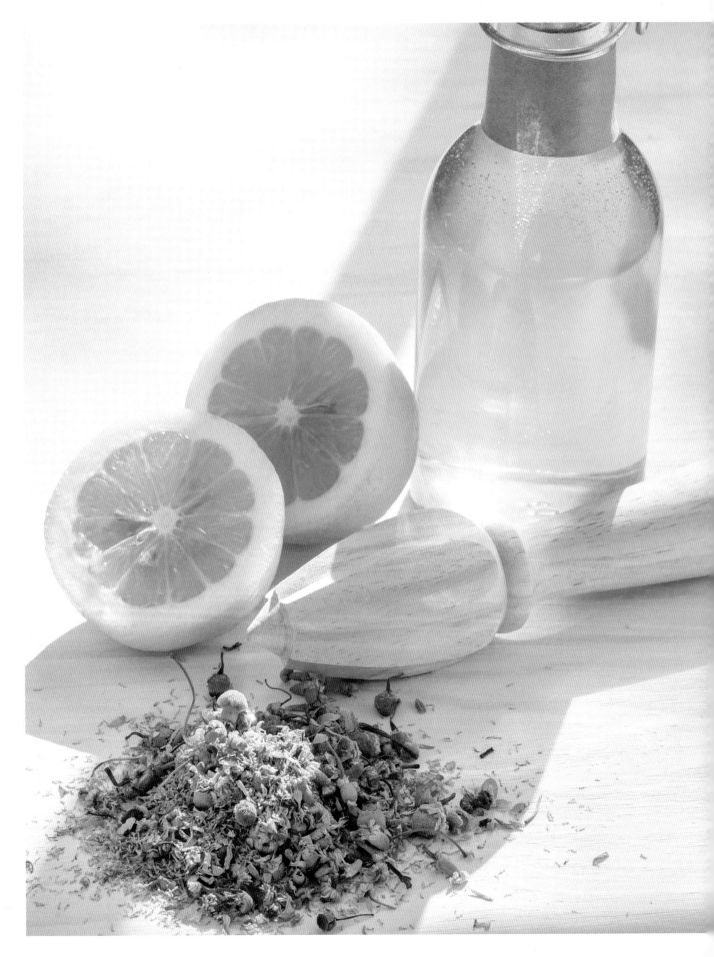

CHAPTER 5

Body Care Recipes

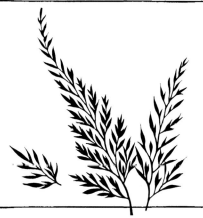

BECAUSE WE TEND TO SPEND MOST OF OUR TIME FOCUSING OUR SKIN CARE EFFORTS ON OUR FACE, WE OFTEN NEGLECT OUR BODIES. FROM SIMPLE EXFOLIATION AND HYDRATION TO INNER HEALTH, THIS CHAPTER FOCUSES ON CARING FOR THE ENTIRE BODY, INSIDE AND OUT. HYDRATING THE SKIN, DE-STRESSING THE BODY, RELAXING THE MIND, AND SOOTHING AN UPSET STOMACH ARE THE JUST A FEW OF THE ESSENTIAL CARE RECIPES YOU'LL SOON LEARN.

Many recipes are given in parts rather than exact measurements; this way you can make as much or as little as desired.

→ ESSENTIAL OILS FOR VARIOUS AILMENTS ←

Here are some important essential oils that are beneficial for different aliments of the body.

★ **Cellulite:** Basil, cypress, fennel, grapefruit, juniper, lavender, lemon, lemongrass, mandarin, pine, and rosemary

★ **Deodorizing:** Bergamot, clary sage, cypress, lavender, patchouli, and tea tree

★ **Sleeplessness:** Basil, chamomile, clary sage, jasmine, lavender, mandarin, rose otto or absolute, and rosewood

★ **Varicose veins:** Cypress, juniper, lavender, and lemon

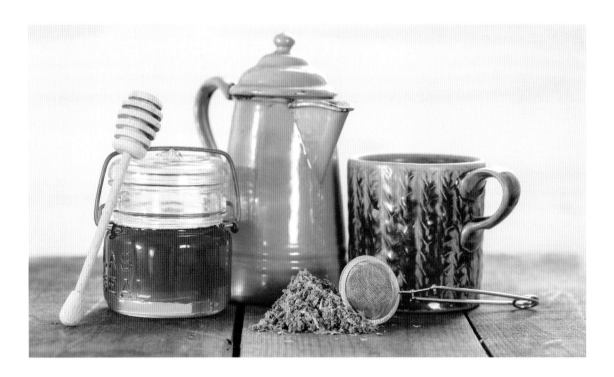

TEAS

Herbal teas, especially for medicinal purposes, have been around for centuries. As discussed in earlier chapters, herbal teas or herbal infusions can be made using dried or fresh leaves, flowers, seeds, or roots of herbs. There are infinite combinations of teas that can be made, whether flavored teas simply for enjoyment or remedy-based recipes. Using the preparation techniques from chapter 3, be creative in your tea mixtures and enjoy.

Sleep Ease Tea

Soothe yourself to sleep with this relaxing blend. Chamomile and valerian are well known for calming the nerves.

INGREDIENTS

1 part chamomile
¼ part oat straw
¼ part linden flower
¼ part dried passionflower leaves
¼ part valerian
¼ part lemon verbena
¼ part calendula
Honey, to taste

DIRECTIONS

Use all the herbs to make an herbal infusion (see page 53).

To use, drink prior to bedtime.

Stress Tea

Fruity and aromatic, chamomile gently calms and lemon balm lifts the spirits and reduces anxiety.

INGREDIENTS

1 part chamomile
$\frac{1}{2}$ part rosehips
$\frac{1}{4}$ part lemon balm
$\frac{1}{4}$ part orange peel
$\frac{1}{4}$ part linden blossoms
$\frac{1}{4}$ part oat straw

DIRECTIONS

Use all the herbs to make an herbal infusion (see page 53).

To use, drink as needed.

Constipation Remedy

Yellow dock is an amazing tonic that gently helps stimulate the digestive system; aided by the other herbs, it makes this a great tea for all your digestive woes.

INGREDIENTS

1 part yellow dock root
$\frac{1}{2}$ part dandelion root
$\frac{1}{2}$ part licorice root
$\frac{1}{4}$ part papaya leaf
$\frac{1}{4}$ part fennel seeds

DIRECTIONS

Use all the herbs to make a decoction (see page 55).

To use, drink 3 or 4 times a day.

Headache Tea

Feverfew is known for its headache- and migraine-alleviating abilities. Lemon balm eases anxiety and calms the nerves.

INGREDIENTS

$\frac{1}{2}$ part lemon balm
$\frac{1}{4}$ part feverfew
$\frac{1}{4}$ part lavender
$\frac{1}{4}$ part chamomile

DIRECTIONS

Use all the herbs to make an herbal infusion (see page 53).

To use, drink as needed, up to 4 or 5 cups a day, until the headache subsides.

Cold Ease Tea

Echinacea is a powerful immune system stimulant, increasing white blood cell production. This tea is great to take with the onset of a cold and has an energizing peppermint flavor.

INGREDIENTS

1 part echinacea root
2 parts peppermint leaves
$\frac{1}{2}$ part yarrow leaves
$\frac{1}{2}$ part lemon balm leaves
$\frac{1}{2}$ part sage leaves
Honey, to taste

DIRECTIONS

Use all the herbs to make an herbal infusion (see page 53).

To use, drink as needed at the onset of a cold.

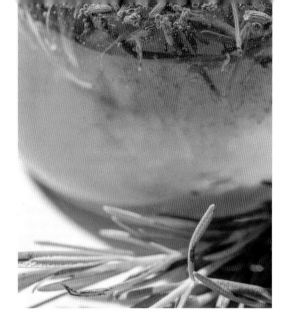

Honey Blends

Honey is often used to promote energy and healing. Internally, mixed with herbs and spices, it is used to treat a variety of ailments. Externally, its naturally humectant and anti-bacterial properties make it valuable in both cosmetics and healing salves or ointments.

Sore Throat and Cough Honey

Use the following herb blend to help soothe a sore throat and ease a cough.

INGREDIENTS

1 part thyme
½ part fenugreek
½ part peppermint
½ part lemon balm

DIRECTIONS

Use all the herbs to make an herbal honey (see page 59).

To use, take 1 to 2 tablespoons (20 to 40 g) daily until symptoms subside. This is also great in tea or warm lemon water.

Cold and Flu Honey

These herbs are known to help fight colds and flu but also help soothe throat and bronchial irritations.

INGREDIENTS

1 part rosemary
1 part elder
½ part ginger
½ part lemon balm

DIRECTIONS

Use all the herbs to make an herbal honey (see page 59).

To use, take 1 to 2 tablespoons (20 to 40 g) daily until symptoms subside. This is also great in tea or warm lemon water.

Stomach Ease

The herbs and spices in this recipe help relieve digestive problems such as nausea and diarrhea. Together they promote healthy digestion.

INGREDIENTS

2 parts papaya leaf
¼ part cinnamon
¼ part turmeric
¼ part cardamom

DIRECTIONS

Use all the herbs to make an herbal honey (see page 59).

To use, take 1 to 2 tablespoons (20 to 40 g) daily until symptoms subside. This is also great in tea or warm lemon water.

TINCTURES

Tincture recipes are great to have on hand, but as you begin to broaden your herbal knowledge you will easily expand you medicine cabinet, too. Tinctures aren't the most palatable because they usually have a very medicinal taste; administration is usually tolerated better by diluting them in water, tea, or juice.

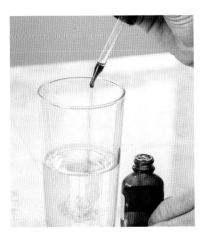

Cold Season Tincture

This blend will ensure a speedy recovery from colds and flu.

INGREDIENTS

1 part thyme leaves
1 part echinacea
1 part violet leaf
1 part peppermint leaf
1 part goldenseal

DIRECTIONS

Use all the herbs to make a tincture (see page 56).

To use, take 3 to 8 drops 2 to 8 times daily until symptoms subside. Can be diluted in water, tea, or juice.

Nerve Tonic Tincture

The herbs used in this blend help calm the nerves, easing anxiety and stress.

INGREDIENTS

1 part chamomile
1 part lemon balm
1 part lavender blossom
2 parts oat straw
¼ part passionflower

DIRECTIONS

Use all the herbs to make a tincture (see page 56).

To use, take 3 to 8 drops 2 to 8 times daily until symptoms subside. Can be diluted in water, tea, or juice.

Skin Blend Tincture

This blend of herbs will help cleanse and beautify the skin from the inside out.

INGREDIENTS

½ part burdock
½ part Oregon grape root
½ part milk thistle
½ part red clover
½ part yellow dock
¼ part thyme leaves

DIRECTIONS

Use all the herbs to make a tincture (see page 56).

To use, take 3 drops daily, morning and night, diluted in water, tea, or juice.

Syrups and Lozenges

A tastier alternative to tinctures, syrups and lozenges make administration, especially to children, a lot easier. See chapter 3 for preparations instructions.

Cough Syrup

This syrup boosts the immune system and soothes bronchial irritation.

INGREDIENTS

$\frac{1}{2}$ cup (16 g) echinacea
$\frac{1}{2}$ cup (16 g) licorice root
2 quarts (2 L) water
2 tablespoons (11 g) ginger root powder
48 ounces (1344 g) organic sugar or
   sweetener of choice

DIRECTIONS

Use all the ingredients to make a syrup (see page 58).

   To use, take 1 to 2 tablespoons (15 to 30 ml) daily until symptoms subside.

Yield: 4 to 6 cups (1 to 1.5 L)

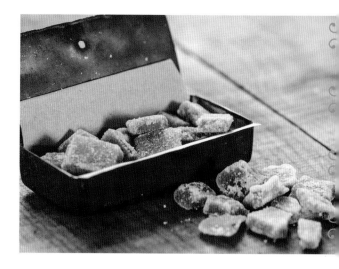

Sore Throat Lozenges

These lozenges are great to soothe an irritated, inflamed throat. I make them every fall and make enough to carry me through the winter. They are a great immune booster to take at the onset of a cold. They freshen the breath, too.

INGREDIENTS

1 ounce (28 g) dried thyme
1 ounce (28 g) dried poplar bud
$\frac{1}{2}$ ounce (14 g) dried echinacea
$\frac{1}{2}$ ounce (14 g) marshmallow
$\frac{1}{4}$ cup (6 g) peppermint leaves
2 cups (470 ml) water
1 tablespoon (8 g) licorice root powder
2 tablespoons (11 g) ginger root powder
2 pounds (905 g) organic sugar
$\frac{1}{2}$ teaspoon cream of tartar
Confectioners' sugar, for sprinkling

DIRECTIONS

Combine the thyme, poplar, echinacea, marshmallow, peppermint, and water in a double boiler. Bring to a simmer (1 & 2).

   Add the licorice and ginger root powders and stir until dissolved (3 & 4). Remove from the heat and strain (5).

Pour the infusion into a saucepan and bring to a boil (6). Add the sugar and cream of tartar (7 & 8). Continue to boil, stirring, until the mixture reaches 265°F (129°C).

Pour the mixture into a well-greased 8 x 11-inch (20.3 x 28 cm) Pyrex dish and set aside to cool (9). Make sure the dish is large enough so the liquid has room to spread and is not too thick. Once the mixture is hard enough to hold its shape, cut it into small pieces (10). Be sure to cut the lozenges before they get too hard or they will break (11).

Lay down waxed paper on your work surface and sprinkle a little confectioners' sugar (alternatively, you could use a little more ginger powder) on it. Break the lozenges up and gently toss in the sugar; this will keep them from sticking together (12). Store in a dry container to use when needed.

Yield: One 8 x 11-inch (20.3 x 28 cm) pan

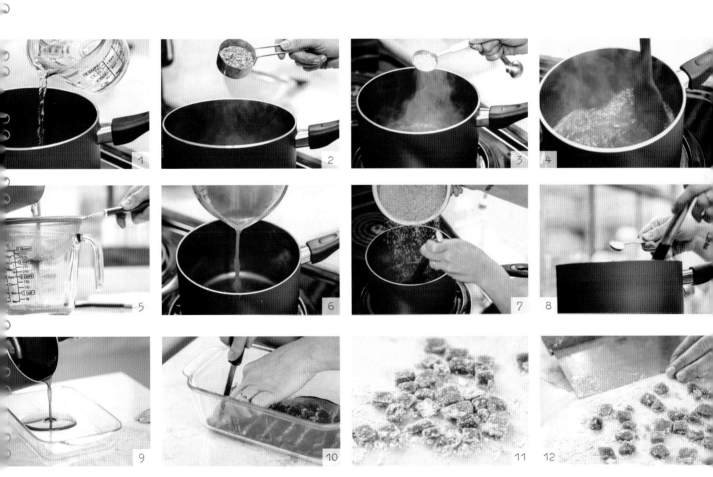

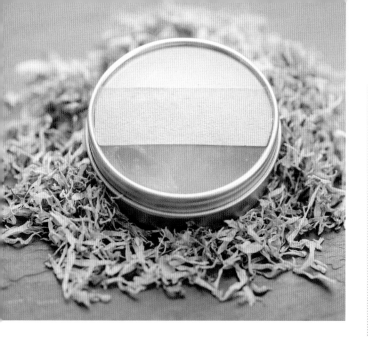

Salves (Ointments)

Salves can be used for a variety of things, from cosmetics to hydrate and fight the signs of aging to treatments to prevent wound infection or ease joint pain. You can adjust the amount of herbs to make a salve of the desired strength. Refer to chapter 3 for preparation instructions.

Calendula and Amaranth Salve for Cuts and Scrapes

Calendula is known for its bacteria-fighting and healing properties. Amaranth flowers, leaves, and roots all possess strong antiseptic properties. This salve is great to use on cuts and scrapes.

INGREDIENTS

2 parts calendula

1 part plantain leaves

1 part amaranth

1 cup (235 ml) oil of choice
  (sesame oil is recommended)

¼ cup (54 g) beeswax

DIRECTIONS

Use all the ingredients to make a salve (see page 60).

To use, apply to cuts and scrapes as needed.

Yield: 1¼ cups (300 ml)

Comfrey Joint and Bruise Salve

Comfrey is highly valued for is soothing abilities, facilitating the healing of damaged tissue.

INGREDIENTS

2 parts comfrey

1 part thyme

1 part rosemary

15 drops arnica extract

5 drops lavender essential oil

1 cup (235 ml) sesame oil or other
  carrier oil of choice

¼ cup (54 g) beeswax

DIRECTIONS

Use all the ingredients to make a salve (see page 60).

To use, apply to the affected area as often as needed.

Yield: 1¼ cups (300 ml)

Beauty Salve

Lavender is known for its amazing hydrating and healing properties when applied to the skin. Hibiscus is beneficial for softening the skin while firming and lifting.

INGREDIENTS

1 part lavender

1 part hibiscus

½ part rose petals

¼ cup (54 g) shea butter

1 cup (235 ml) jojoba or rosehip oil

¼ cup (54 g) beeswax

DIRECTIONS

Use all the ingredients to make a salve (see page 60).

To use, apply daily to face or to areas of concern, such as the lips, under the eyes, or the neck. This can even be used as a cuticle treatment or on the elbows and heels.

Yield: 1¼ cups (300 ml)

POULTICES AND COMPRESSES

A great technique for treating skin aliments like breakouts, cuts, and bruises is to use a poultice. Poultices are an herbal blend in oil or water to create a paste. They can then be applied as is to an area for treatment, or they can be spread on gauze or muslin to create a compress that can be applied to or wrapped around the affected area for an extended period of time.

Wound Healing Poultice and Compress

This is a great poultice for infected or slow to heal skin sores.

INGREDIENTS

2 tablespoons (12 g) fresh calendula, or 1 tablespoon (1.6 g) dried

2 tablespoons (12 g) fresh comfrey, or 1 tablespoon (1.6 g) dried

1 tablespoon (15 ml) warm water

5 drops lavender essential oil

DIRECTIONS

In a mortar and pestle, combine the herbs and water. Mash together to create a poultice. Add the essential oil and mix well.

To use, scoop the mixture onto a strip of gauze and layer another strip of gauze over the top. Wrap the compress around the affected area and let sit for at least 20 to 40 minutes. Can be reapplied as needed.

Yield: 1 poultice

Varicose Veins Poultice and Compress

Yarrow, a natural anti-inflammatory, helps tone varicose veins.

INGREDIENTS

2 tablespoons (12 g) yarrow

1 tablespoon (15 ml) warm water

5 drops cypress essential oil

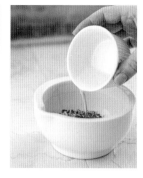
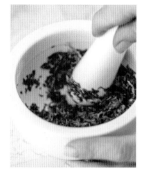

DIRECTIONS

In a mortar and pestle, combine the yarrow and water. Mash together to create a poultice. Add the essential oil and mix well.

To use, scoop the mixture onto a strip of gauze and layer another strip of gauze over the top. Wrap the compress around the affected area and let sit for at least 20 to 40 minutes. Can be reapplied as needed.

Yield: 1 poultice

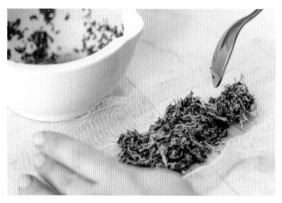

Sprain Poultice and Compress

Yarrow works as an anti-inflammatory, and horsetail, with its high mineral content, helps heal bones and joints.

INGREDIENTS

2 tablespoons (12 g) comfrey
1 tablespoon (6 g) horsetail
1 tablespoon (15 ml) warm water
5 drops lavender essential oil

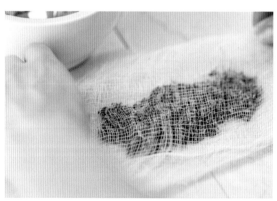

DIRECTIONS

In a mortar and pestle, combine the yarrow, horsetail, and water. Mash together to create a poultice. Add the essential oil and mix well.

To use, scoop the mixture onto a strip of gauze and layer another strip of gauze over the top. Wrap the compress around the affected area and let sit for at least 20 to 40 minutes. Can be reapplied as needed.

Yield: 1 poultice

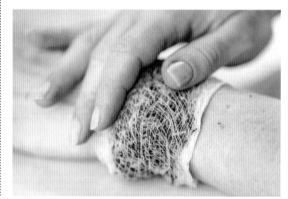

To create a compress, mash the ingredients together, place the mixture between layers of gauze, and apply to the affected area.

Steam Inhalations

Steams are not only beneficial for the external health of the skin, but they can also be a great medicinal aid during cold season to help with sinus infections and congestion. (Steams are not recommended for weeping acne or sensitive, sunburned, or damaged skin.)

Congestion Relief Steam

This steam works double-time to clear not only the skin but also the sinuses from congestion.

INGREDIENTS

2 quarts (2 L) distilled water
3 tablespoons (18 g) eucalyptus leaves
1 tablespoon (2.5 g) sage leaves
1 tablespoon (6 g) ginkgo biloba leaves
1 tablespoon (1.7 g) rosemary leaves
2 drops clove essential oil
2 drops clove juniper essential oil
2 drops ravensara essential oil

DIRECTIONS

Bring the water to a boil in a teakettle. Pour it into a bowl, add the herbs and essential oils, and let steep for a few minutes.

To use, place the bowl in an area where you can comfortably sit while leaning over for at least 10 minutes. Using a towel, create a tent over your head, place your face over the steam, and take calming deep breaths.

Yield: 1 steam

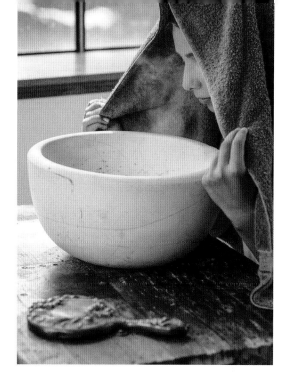

Pore-Refining Steam

This steam unclogs the pores and leaves the skin refreshed and moisturized.

INGREDIENTS

3 cups (705 ml) distilled water
¼ cup (60 ml) apple cider vinegar
1 teaspoon lavender
1 teaspoon rosemary
1 teaspoon chamomile

DIRECTIONS

Bring the water to a boil in a teakettle. Pour it into a bowl, add the vinegar and herbs, and let steep for a few minutes.

To use, place the bowl in an area where you can comfortably sit while leaning over for at least 10 minutes. Using a towel, create a tent over your head and place your face over the steam.

Yield: 1 steam

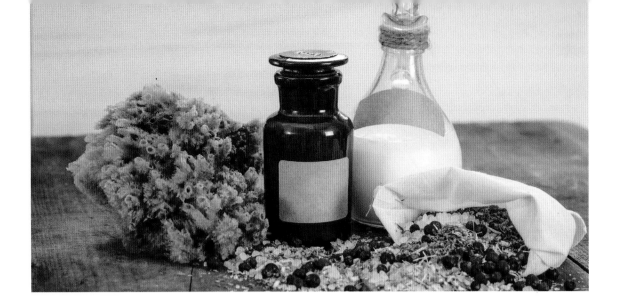

Bath Soaks

When used in the bath, salts and herbs can help alleviate many ailments, from sore muscles and joints to stress and dry skin.

Joint and Muscle Soak

This detoxifying soak will soothe and relax achy joints and muscles.

INGREDIENTS

1 cup (288 g) Epsom salt
¼ cup (72 g) dendrite salt
½ cup (120 g) baking soda
¼ cup (24 g) juniper berries
3 drops cypress essential oil
3 drops peppermint essential oil
3 drops chamomile essential oil
3 drops rosemary essential oil

DIRECTIONS

Gather all the ingredients and put in a muslin bag, shake it, and tie it shut.

To use, place the bag in the tub under warm running water. The bag can remain in the tub throughout your entire bath.

Yield: 1 bath bag

Relaxing Bath Bag

Wash the day's stresses away with this amazing blend of herbs geared to ease tension and stress.

INGREDIENTS

¼ cup (8 g) dried chamomile
¼ cup (8 g) dried lavender
¼ cup (8 g) dried rose hips
1 tablespoon (8 g) dried comfrey leaf

DIRECTIONS

Gather all the ingredients and put in a muslin bag, shake it, and tie it shut.

To use, place the bag in the tub under warm running water. Relax and soak. The bag can remain in the tub throughout your entire bath.

Yield: 1 bath bag

Cold and Flu Bath Oil

An oil bath not only eases sore muscles and aches associated with a cold or flu, but it also offers aromatherapy to ease congestion.

INGREDIENTS

2 tablespoons (30 ml) jojoba oil
2 tablespoons (30 ml) sweet almond oil
3 drops sweet basil essential oil
3 drops rosemary essential oil
3 drops peppermint essential oil
3 drops eucalyptus essential oil
3 drops lemon essential oil

DIRECTIONS

Add all the oils to warm running bathwater and stir. Relax and soak.

Yield: 1 bath

Skin-Softening Milk Bath

This bath treatment relieves stress, eases aches and pains, and softens the skin.

INGREDIENTS

1/2 cup (144 g) Epsom salt
1/4 cup (60 g) baking soda
1/4 cup (60 ml) coconut milk
2 tablespoons (30 ml) sweet almond oil
2 drops vanilla extract
3 drops geranium essential oil
3 drops chamomile essential oil
2 drops clary sage essential oil

DIRECTIONS

Add all the ingredients to warm running bathwater and stir. Relax and soak.

Yield: 1 bath

Footbath

This refreshing recipe moisturizes and softens tired, overworked feet.

INGREDIENTS

5 to 6 cups (1175 to 1410 ml) boiling
  water
1/2 cup (16 g) dried lavender
1/4 cup (22 g) dried ginger or ginger
  powder
1/4 cup (8 g) ground sage
2 tablespoons (3 g) dried peppermint
2 tablespoons (7 g) dried rosemary
10 drops lemon verbena essential oil
1 tablespoon (20 g) Epsom salt

DIRECTIONS

Combine all the ingredients in a large bowl or footbath. Let steep until cool enough to be tolerated by your feet.

To use, soak your feet and relax. Always be sure to test the water before putting your feet in.

Yield: 1 footbath

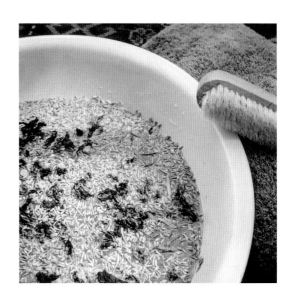

Body Butters and Scrubs

Body butters are thick creams made with active ingredients that are known for their healing and moisturizing effects. Body scrubs can be made using a variety of exfoliating ingredients that help slough away dead skin cells, revealing healthy skin and allowing for better penetration of lotions and creams.

Intense Moisture Body Butter

This recipe is a simple yet extremely moisturizing body butter that will handle even the driest of skin. The following oils are known for their moisturizing abilities, but feel free to experiment with any oils you love.

INGREDIENTS
2 tablespoons (28 g) cocoa butter
2 tablespoons (28 g) shea butter
1 tablespoon (15 ml) buriti fruit oil
1 tablespoon (15 ml) sweet almond oil
1 tablespoon (15 ml) meadowfoam seed oil
1 tablespoon (15 ml) avocado oil
1 tablespoon (15 ml) coconut oil
2 tablespoons (28 g) beeswax

DIRECTIONS
Melt all the ingredients together in a double boiler until well blended, stirring frequently. Pour the mixture into a sterile, sealable container and let it cool. This recipe will keep for a month when stored in proper container and kept in a cool area.

To use, apply the butter to elbows, heels, or any other areas in need of extreme moisture.

Yield: 2/3 cup (165 g)

Coconut Balm

This balm is extremely moisturizing, and it smells great, too.

INGREDIENTS
7 tablespoons (105 ml) coconut oil
1 tablespoon (14 g) cocoa butter
1½ teaspoons shea butter
1 teaspoon beeswax
15 drops sweet orange essential oil
5 drops ginger essential oil

DIRECTIONS
Melt all the ingredients together in a double boiler until well blended, stirring frequently. Pour the mixture into a sterile, sealable container and let it cool.

To use, rub on areas of the body that need the most moisture. Apply as needed.

Yield: 1/2 cup (120 ml)

Coconut Brown Sugar Body Scrub

A great summertime exfoliant, this scrub leaves the skin smooth, hydrated, and smelling wonderful.

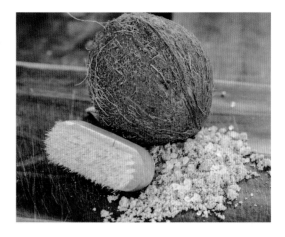

INGREDIENTS

6 tablespoons (90 ml) coconut oil

1 cup (225 g) packed coarse brown sugar

5 drops ginger essential oil

DIRECTIONS

In a double boiler, melt the coconut oil (if needed), and then add the sugar and essential oil, mixing well. Pour the mixture into a sterile, sealable container and let it cool.

To use, while in the shower, rub the scrub in gentle circular motions using your hand, a washcloth, or a loofah. Rinse and pat dry.

Yield: 1 ⅓ cups (315 g)

Cellulite Body Scrub

This recipe combines all the cellulite-fighting ingredients I love into one amazing scrub. Although it is not the prettiest product, it's definitely effective with continued use.

INGREDIENTS

⅓ cup (40 g) powdered kelp

¼ cup (20 g) dulse

¼ cup (50 g) sugar

½ cup (60 g) freshly ground coffee beans

¼ cups (80 g) coarse sea salt

1 cup (235 ml) sesame oil (other oils of your choice can be substituted; sweet almond oil works well, too)

10 drops grapefruit essential oil

DIRECTIONS

Mix all the ingredients together and pour into a sterile container of your choice. This recipe can be doubled and stored in the refrigerator for up to 2 or 3 weeks.

To use, while in shower, using your fingertips or a loofah sponge, apply the mixture to the thigh area or any other areas affected by cellulite, and massage thoroughly.

Yield: 2 cups (470 ml)

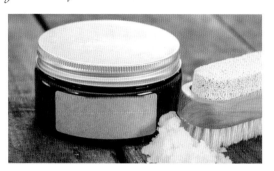

Brown Sugar Foot Scrub

This recipe is great for exfoliating and moisturizing dry, cracked feet.

INGREDIENTS

1 teaspoon coconut oil

¼ cup (60 g) brown sugar

2 tablespoons (30 ml) freshly squeezed lemon juice

2 tablespoons aloe vera juice

DIRECTIONS

In a sterile, microwavable container, melt the coconut oil and then stir in the sugar, lemon juice, and aloe vera, mixing well.

To use, take about a tablespoon (15 ml), or more if desired, per foot, and using either your hand or a foot brush, rub the heels and undersides of your feet. Rinse with water and pat dry.

Yield: ¼ cup (60 g)

Pumice Foot Scrub

This foot scrub recipe is also great for exfoliating and moisturizing dry, cracked feet, but it uses pumice stone instead of brown sugar.

INGREDIENTS

2 tablespoons (15 g) ground pumice powder

¼ cup (60 ml) sesame oil

10 drops eucalyptus essential oil

DIRECTIONS

In a sterile container, combine all the ingredients and mix well.

To use, take about a tablespoon (15 ml), or more if desired, per foot, and using either your hand or foot brush, rub the heels and undersides of your feet. Rinse with water and pat dry.

Yield: ¼ cup (60 g)

MASSAGE OILS

Massage oils are always great to have on hand for both you and your partner. Massage is a great way to relieve stress, release toxins, and ease sore muscles. Always be sure to drink plenty of water with lemon after a massage to help flush all the toxins out of your body.

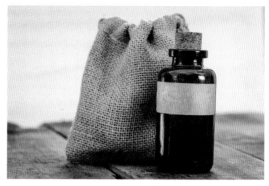

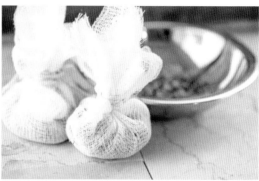

Couples Massage Oil

Here's a great way to show someone he or she is appreciated. A mix of cinnamon essential oil and vanilla extract are both comforting and intoxicating. Cinnamon has a warming effect and has long been used in love potions. Vanilla exudes a sense of calm and comfort.

INGREDIENTS

1 cup (235 ml) grapeseed oil

¼ cup (60 ml) wheat germ oil

10 drops cinnamon essential oil

5 drops vanilla extract

DIRECTIONS

In a sterile container, combine all the ingredients and mix well. This mixture will keep for 3 to 6 months when stored correctly.

To use, massage the oil in gentle circles on skin as needed.

Yield: 1¼ cups (295 ml)

Massage Poultice

A favorite relaxing massage treatment is a massage poultice, which relieves stress and relaxes sore muscles. This can be made with any combination of herbs; feel free to experiment with different oils, which help hydrate and soothe the skin. For really sore or bruised muscles, add a few drops of arnica essential oil. Both your skin and your muscles will feel like they spent the day at the spa.

INGREDIENTS

½ cup (120 ml) almond oil

2 tablespoons (30 ml) coconut oil

3 tablespoons (6 g) dried lavender

3 tablespoons (6 g) dried jasmine

1 tablespoon (6 g) juniper berries

3 tablespoons (10 g) dried rosemary

DIRECTIONS

In a double boiler, heat the almond oil and coconut oil until both are warm (1). Do not let them get too hot.

Mix the dried herbs together and divide in half; put each half in the center of a piece of muslin or cheesecloth (2). Gather the sides of the cloth and tie together with kitchen twine (3 & 4).

Place both bags in the oil and let them sit until they are fully saturated (5).

Test to make sure the oil isn't too hot before using it for massage. To use, massage the poultices in gentle circular motions on the affected area (6). When the poultices cool off, place them back in the oil until they are warm again, remembering to always check the temperature before beginning the massage.

Yield: 2 poultices

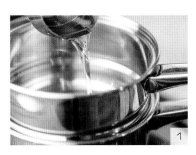
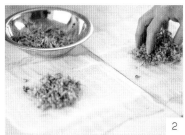
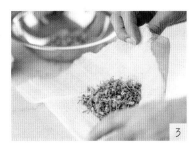
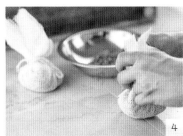
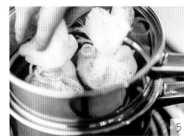
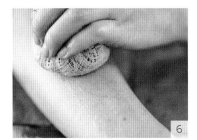

Sore Muscle Massage Oil

Relieve aching muscles and joints with this blend of powerful oils.

INGREDIENTS

1 cup (235 ml) grapeseed oil
¼ cup (60 ml) wheat germ oil
1 tablespoon (15 ml) arnica oil
15 drops camphor essential oil
15 drops cypress essential oil

DIRECTIONS

In a sterile container, combine all the ingredients and mix well. This mixture will keep for 3 to 6 months when stored correctly. To make this massage oil extra effective, you can heat the grapeseed oil in a double boiler over low heat for 15 to 20 minutes with ¼ cup (24 g) of juniper berries. Strain the juniper berries and add the remainder of the ingredients for a warm, relaxing muscle massage.

To use, massage the oil in gentle circles on skin as needed. If you are using heated oil, be sure to test the temperature before applying to the skin.

Yield: 1¼ cups (295 ml)

BODY POWDERS AND DEODORANTS

Body powders are a blend of different powders that have beneficial properties for the skin and absorb odor and oils. Deodorants help absorb and fight odor-causing bacteria, leaving a fresh scent.

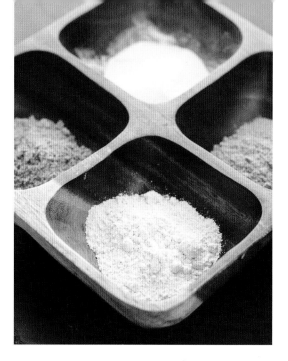

Body Powder

A refreshing blend of powders absorbs moisture while leaving behind a light lavender scent.

INGREDIENTS

1 cup (120 g) kaolin clay
1 cup (120 g) arrowroot powder
½ cup (60 g) rice flour
¼ cup (30 g) lavender powder
10 drops essential oil of your choice

DIRECTIONS

Combine the clay, arrowroot powder, flour, and lavender powder in a bowl. While stirring, slowly add the essential oil drop by drop, making sure it is evenly distributed throughout.

To use, apply to the body as needed.

Yield: 2¾ cups (330 g)

Foot Powder

Moisture absorbing and odor blocking, this powder is great for the feet.

INGREDIENTS

1 cup (220 g) baking soda
1 cup (120 g) arrowroot powder
¼ cup (30 g) powdered orange peel
  (if available)
25 drops peppermint essential oil
15 drops tea tree essential oil

DIRECTIONS

Combine all the powders in a bowl. While mixing, slowly add the essential oils drop by drop, making sure they are evenly distributed.

To use, sprinkle the desired amount directly onto the feet or into socks or shoes.

Yield: 2 ¼ cups (370 g)

Deodorant Cream

The powerful odor-absorbing properties of baking soda, geranium, tea tree essential oil, and hydrating coconut oil will make this deodorant a favorite.

INGREDIENTS

1 tablespoon (14 g) beeswax
1 tablespoon (14 g) candelilla wax
¼ cup (60 ml) coconut oil
2 tablespoons (30 ml) jojoba oil
2 tablespoons (28 g) baking soda
1 tablespoon (8 g) arrowroot powder
1 tablespoon (8 g) kaolin clay
10 drops geranium essential oil
10 drops tea tree essential oil
Optional deodorizing essential oils:
  Geranium, lemon, tea tree, lavender,
  cypress

DIRECTIONS

In a double boiler, melt the waxes, coconut oil, and jojoba oil, stirring to combine (1). Pour into a clean glass bowl or measuring cup (2).

Add the baking soda, arrowroot powder, and clay and mix well (3). Then add the essential oils drop by drop and mix until blended (4).

Pour the mixture into a clean container or roll-up stick (5 & 6).

To use, apply as needed.

Yield: ¾ cup (160 g)

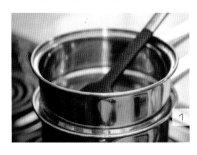
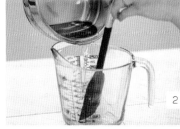
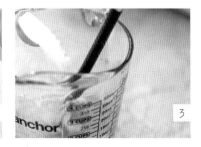
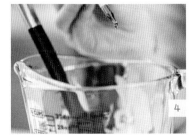
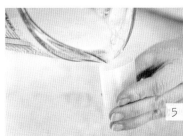
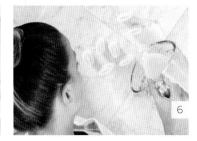

Toothpastes

Both of these toothpaste recipes are a great way to save some money while effectively cleaning your teeth. Baking soda has been used in dental care extensively, and both peppermint and cinnamon freshen the breath. Either of these recipes can be made ahead of time in larger batches for daily use; just don't add the oil (in the first recipe) or water (in the second) until you're ready to brush. The teeth-whitening treatment is also an inexpensive way to remove stains.

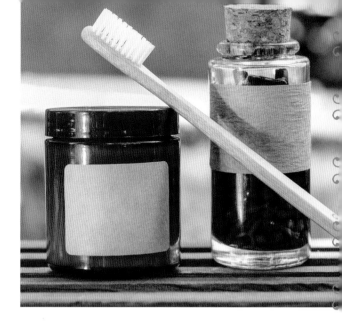

Peppermint Toothpaste

Peppermint's antiseptic properties help rid the mouth of harmful, toothache-causing bacteria while freshening the breath.

INGREDIENTS

1½ teaspoons dried peppermint leaves

½ cup (120 ml) distilled water

½ teaspoon sweet almond oil

½ teaspoon cornstarch

DIRECTIONS

Make an herbal infusion using the peppermint leaves and distilled water (see page 53), and then store in a separate sealable container (this can also double as a mouthwash).

To use, in a small bowl, mix the oil and cornstarch to create a paste, place on your toothbrush, and pour a small amount of the infusion over the toothbrush. Brush as usual.

Yield: ½ cup (120 ml)

Cinnamon Toothpaste

Cinnamon has both antiseptic and astringent properties, ridding bacteria and freshening the breath, making it a great choice for use in toothpastes and mouthwashes.

INGREDIENTS

1 tablespoon (14 g) baking soda

1 teaspoon ground cinnamon

½ cup (120 ml) distilled water

DIRECTIONS

Mix the baking soda and cinnamon together in a small bowl, and then add the water to create a paste.

To use, apply the paste to a toothbrush and brush as usual.

Yield: ½ cup (120 ml)

Strawberry Teeth-Whitening Treatment

This is a great treatment to help whiten teeth.

INGREDIENTS

3 large strawberries
2 teaspoons baking soda
½ teaspoon cream of tartar
1 cup (235 ml) distilled water
¼ teaspoon salt

DIRECTIONS

Purée the strawberries in a blender or food processor. Set aside. Combine the baking soda and cream of tartar in a small bowl, then add some water to create a paste. Set aside. Add the salt to the remaining water in a glass.

To use, gently brush the purée onto the teeth. Let sit for at least 5 minutes. Next, gently brush the paste onto the teeth. Finally, rinse with the salt water. This treatment should be done no more than once a week.

Yield: 1 treatment

MOUTHWASHES

Both of these mouthwashes are refreshing and cleansing; the alcohol helps kill bacteria, so they can be made in larger quantities.

Apple and Clove Mouthwash

Clove is a natural antiseptic that kills harmful bacteria, and it also contains analgesic properties, which can help the pain of toothaches.

INGREDIENTS

¼ cup (60 ml) vodka
½ cup (120 ml) distilled water
15 drops clove essential oil
10 drops mint essential oil
1 teaspoon organic no-sugar-added
   apple juice

DIRECTIONS

In a sterile sealable container, combine all the ingredients

To use, swish about 2 tablespoons (30 ml) of the mouthwash for at least 30 seconds before spitting out.

Yield: ¾ cup (180 ml)

Cinnamon and Tea Tree Mouthwash

This mouthwash can also be poured onto a cotton ball and placed over the affected tooth to kill bacteria and ease pain.

INGREDIENTS

1 cinnamon stick
1 tablespoon (5 g) whole cloves
1 cup (235 ml) vodka
5 drops tea tree essential oil

DIRECTIONS

Make a tincture using the cinnamon, cloves, and vodka (see page 56). Once the tincture is ready, add the tea tree oil and pour into a sterile sealable container.

To use, swish about 2 tablespoons (30 ml) of mouthwash for at least 30 seconds before spitting out.

Yield: 1 cup (235 ml)

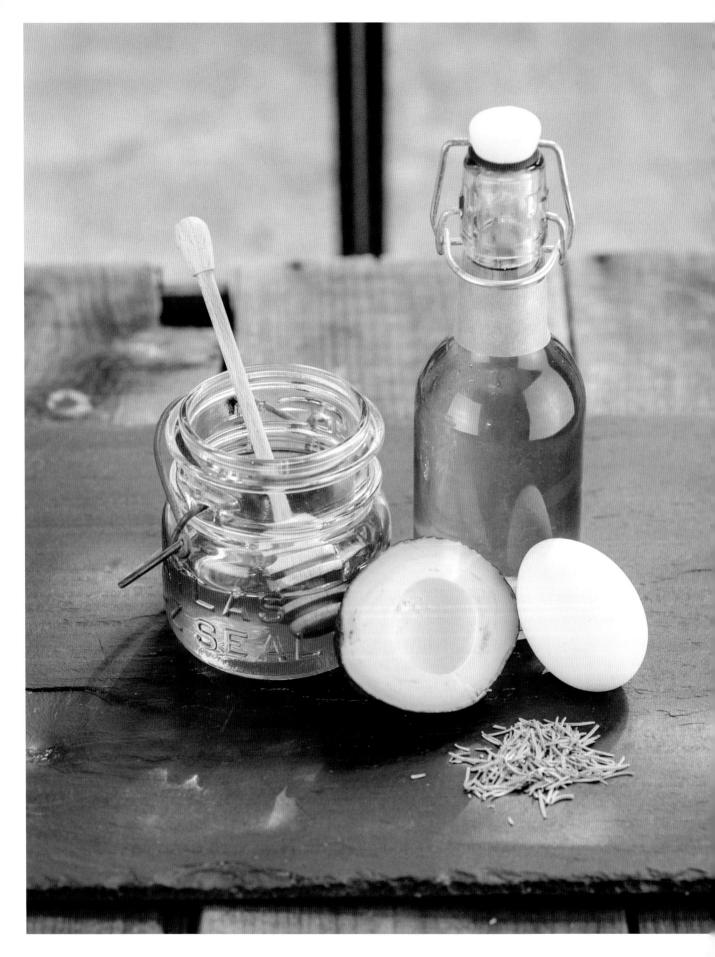

CHAPTER 6

Hair Care Recipes

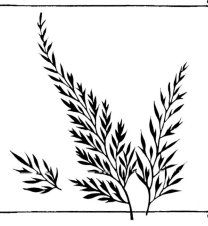

Taking care of your hair and scalp are essential for overall optimal health. This chapter will teach you not only the essentials to taking care of your hair but also how to make everything you'll need.

→ KITCHEN RESCUES ←

Here are some quick hair rescues that you'll find in your kitchen.

★ **Apple cider vinegar:** Adds shine and cleans and restores health to the scalp.

★ **Avocado oil:** Rich in protein, it restores health to hair and reduces frizz.

★ **Beer:** Full of yeast, beer naturally plumps fine limp hair.

★ **Egg:** Rich in fats and proteins, it moisturizes and removes oils.

★ **Honey:** A natural humectant, honey moisturizes and restores health to damaged hair.

★ **Rosemary:** Create an infusion for dry hair and scalp.

★ **Yogurt or sour cream:** Lactic acid works great on dull hair, removing residue and restoring shine.

HAIR CARE 101

If you're like most people, your hair suffers a continual beating. From the everyday environmental damaging effects to those we bring on ourselves with chemical treatments and blow-drying, it's no wonder people are forever on the hunt for some miracle hair product. Hate to break the bad news to you, but there is no one product that will solve all your hair's woes, regardless of its claims. The further your hair grows out from the scalp, the more prone it is to becoming dry and damaged, because it is no longer living, but just a protein. Your scalp produces oil as part of our body's natural cleansing and moisturizing defense. With a healthy diet and hair care regimen, you can very easily keep your hair healthy and manageable. Understanding what you can and cannot control when it comes to your hair is key to maintaining healthy hair.

Your hair care regimen should consist of the following: shampoo, conditioner, and weekly conditioning treatments. With that said, let's discuss shampoo.

While keeping clean is essential to a healthy scalp (and thus healthy hair), it is not true that your hair needs to be washed every day. Depending on your hair type, you may be able to extend the length of time in between washings. Why not wash? Well, it's simple: your scalp is an extension of your face. Skin is skin, after all, and your scalp is still part of that largest organ system we discussed earlier. The more you wash it, the drier it becomes, just like your face. And just like your face, the more you wash it, drying it out, the more your body's natural defense system kicks in to produce more oils to moisturize it.

So a good gentle, nondrying shampoo is the most important part of hair care, not conditioner, which is often the belief. Think of shampoo as your foundation: if you don't start with a healthy, moisture-rich foundation, no matter how good the conditioner may claim to be, it will never completely restore the damage done by a bad shampoo. Yes, all the hype you've heard about drying sulfates and chemicals in shampoo is true, and yes there is some truth to the belief that the less you wash, the less oils your scalp will naturally produce.

Most people, especially those with finer hair who insist on daily washing, receive this advice with much skepticism. I do promise this: using a gentle, sulfate-free, nondrying shampoo no more than every other day will eventually reduce oil production. While this may take several weeks to a month to reset itself from years of overproduction to counteract continual stripping, it will in fact do just that.

In the meantime, there are numerous dry shampoos that work great for refreshing and absorbing oils in between washings. Or if you really must, you can wet your hair every day and go through the motions of shampooing, using your natural oils as a cleanser. Just keep in mind that if this daily wetting is only followed by the drying effects of blow-drying and straightening, you're not helping yourself any. In the end, though, as long as you are using a high-quality, nondrying shampoo, you're okay. However, selecting a shampoo that's right for your hair is key.

Dry Hair		Normal Hair		Oily Hair		To Add Shine		Dandruff Remedies		Thinning and Volume
Avocado oil, elderflower, yarrow, chamomile, comfrey root		Horsetail, dandelion, clover		Watercress, lemongrass, white willow bark, clary sage		Apple cider vinegar, egg, nettle, raspberry		Apple cider vinegar, white willow bark, nettle, peppermint		Watercress, apple cider vinegar, nettle, sage, basil, rosemary, licorice

Another important thing to keep in mind regarding shampoo is that it should only be applied from the nape up. The ends of your hair (the quickest to dry and split) don't need shampoo; they will get enough cleansing when you rinse. And no, your shampoo doesn't need to lather in order to work. In fact, often greasy, dirtier hair will lather less than clean hair anyway. To explain the way shampoo functions regardless of its lather content, without getting too chemistry teacher on you, consider this: the main components of shampoo (or any detergent or soap) have two ends, your oil-loving end (lipophilic) and your water-loving end (hydrophilic). The oil-loving end naturally attaches itself to the oils and residue in your hair. During the rinsing/wetting process, the water-loving end attaches to the water, and this motion between the two ends creates a lather. So as you can see, the lather is not as essential to the cleansing action as we may believe it is.

Conditioner, meanwhile, is an essential component of a healthy hair care regimen. Your hair, depending on length, is for the most part just dead protein, and therefore retaining as much moisture as possible is key. Using a daily hydrating conditioner that doesn't weigh your hair down is vital to hair and scalp health, along with a weekly deep conditioning mask. Applying conditioner to only the body and ends of the hair will avoid weighing it down and making the scalp look greasier.

And we have some hair care myths to dispel. The first myth: split ends can be repaired. No matter what the product claims, this is just simply not true. Although it might mask the damage or smooth the flyaways, that is where it ends. Most of these products are laden with silicones that build up in the hair, damaging it even more, not to mention their health and environmental concerns. Again, the ends of your hair are dead proteins, and once they split there is no bringing them back to life. Frequent trims are the only sure way to rid your hair of split ends.

Another myth to lay to rest is the idea that frequently changing your shampoo keeps your hair from getting used to it; this is simply not true. As long as you are using a healthy shampoo suited for your hair type, change isn't necessary.

Shampoos and Rinses

The great thing about making your own shampoo is that you can customize it to meet your hair's needs. If you tend to have naturally greasier hair, use shampoos geared toward reducing oil production. If your hair is dry, use shampoos that use hydrating oils to cleanse.

Shampoo Rinse

This easy at-home shampoo uses any unscented liquid castile soap you prefer. This recipe is easily customized to your particular hair type or need.

INGREDIENTS

¼ cup (60 ml) herbal infusion for your hair type (see page 127)
½ cup (120 ml) liquid castile soap
2 tablespoons (30 ml) aloe vera juice
5 drops grapefruit seed extract
10 drops essential oil for your hair type (see page 127)

DIRECTIONS

Once you have made your infusion (see page 53), add the rest of the ingredients, mix well, and pour into a sterile bottle.

To use, apply to hair and shampoo as usual. Rinse and follow with conditioner.

Yield: ¾ cup (180 ml)

Clarifying Shampoo

This recipe is great for oily hair, dry scalp, or to remove buildup and restore shine.

INGREDIENTS

1½ teaspoons dried lavender
1½ teaspoons dried rosemary
1½ teaspoons dried basil
½ cup (120 ml) distilled water
1 cup (235 ml) liquid castile soap
¼ cup (60 ml) apple cider vinegar
2 tablespoon (30 ml) jojoba oil
5 drops lemon essential oil
5 drops thyme essential oil
2 drops cypress essential oil

DIRECTIONS

Make an infusion using the herbs and water (see page 53). Combine the rest of the ingredients in a separate container, add ½ cup (120 ml) of the herbal infusion, and mix well. Pour into a sterile bottle.

To use, shampoo as usual. Rinse and follow with conditioner.

Yield: 2 cups (470 ml)

Dandruff Rinse

Great for dry, itchy scalp relief, this rinse can be used twice a week to heal the scalp and remove flakiness.

INGREDIENTS

1½ teaspoons fresh lemongrass
1½ teaspoons peppermint
1½ teaspoons horsetail
1½ teaspoons nettle
1½ teaspoons rosemary
1½ teaspoons tea tree leaf
2 cups (470 ml) distilled water
¼ cup (60 ml) apple cider vinegar

DIRECTIONS

Make an infusion with the herbs and water (see page 53), and then add the apple cider vinegar to the infusion. Pour into a sterile bottle.

To use, after your regular shampoo, apply the rinse and leave it on for at least a minute, then rinse. Follow with conditioner applied from the nape down. Repeat this rinse at least two times a week until condition improves.

Yield: 2 cups (470 ml)

Quick Refreshing Hair Rinse

This is a refreshing rinse for both the scalp and the hair. It's easy to make, and you can use either a mint tea or fresh mint leaves for the infusion. This rinse is great for removing smoke and other environmental odors from the hair.

INGREDIENTS

1 cup (235 ml) mint herbal infusion (see page 53)
2 tablespoons (30 ml) apple cider vinegar

DIRECTIONS

Combine the herbal infusion and add the apple cider vinegar to the infusion. Pour into a sterile bottle.

To use, after your regular shampoo, apply the rinse and leave on for at least a minute, then rinse. Follow with conditioner.

Yield: 1 cup (235 ml)

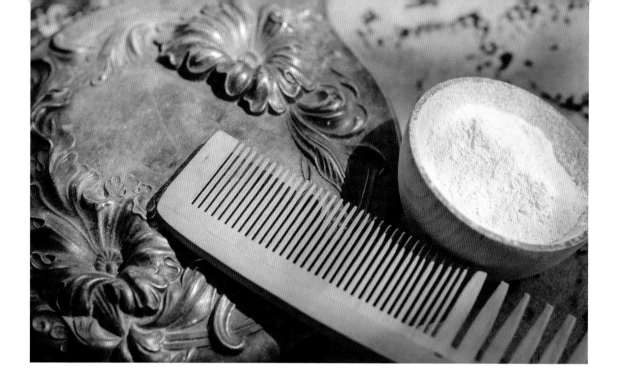

Dry Shampoo

This is a great alternative to the traditionally wet shampoo. It's perfect for those on the go or as a refresher in between shampoos.

INGREDIENTS

½ cup (120 g) rice flour
¼ cup (56 g) baking soda
¼ cup (30 g) powdered orange peel
5 drops patchouli essential oil

DIRECTIONS

Combine the flour, baking soda, and powdered orange peel in a bowl, mix well, and continue stirring as you slowly add the essential oil until fully blended. Pour into a sterile bottle.

To use, sprinkle a little of the powder into your hair. Then work it into the scalp until it is absorbed.

Yield: 1 cup (200 g)

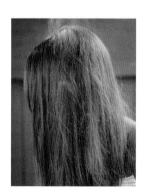
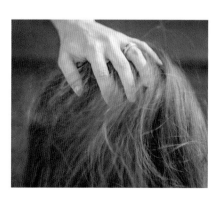
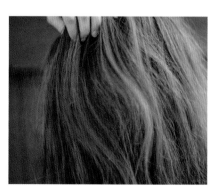

CONDITIONERS AND TREATMENT OILS

Conditioner plays an important role in keeping hair smooth, shiny, and healthy, replacing the sebum (your natural oils) that is lost from your hair after shampooing. However, overdoing conditioning can end up making your hair dull and lifeless. So only condition when needed. The recipes below are great conditioning treatments that can be used once or twice a week to maintain hair health without weighing it down or building up residue.

Hair Conditioning Mask

Natural moisturizing oils treat overly dry, porous hair, restoring luster and shine.

INGREDIENTS
1 tablespoon (15 ml) jojoba oil
1 teaspoon sweet almond oil
1 teaspoon avocado oil
1 teaspoon olive oil
1 egg yolk
1 tablespoon (20 g) honey

DIRECTIONS
Combine all the ingredients until well blended.

To use, apply to damp hair and work through. Wrap hair in a plastic shower cap and let the mixture sit for 20 minutes. Then rinse, shampoo, and condition as usual.

Yield: 1 hair mask

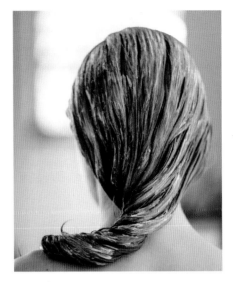
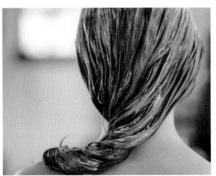
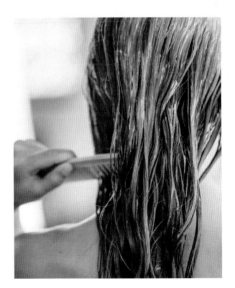

Leave-in Hair Oil and Frizz Tamer

A great treatment for overly dry, processed hair, this oil blend hydrates and smoothes the hair, giving it shine and fighting flyaways. It leaves the hair smelling great, too.

INGREDIENTS

3 tablespoons (30 ml) avocado oil
3 tablespoons (30 ml) jojoba oil
½ teaspoon coconut oil
3 drops geranium essential oil
3 drops lavender essential oil
3 drops rosemary essential oil

DIRECTIONS

In a double boiler over low heat, melt the avocado, jojoba, and coconut oils together until blended. Remove from the heat and allow to cool before adding the essential oils. Stored in a sterile container away from heat and direct sunlight, this oil will keep for 3 to 4 months.

To use, apply a small amount to your fingertips and gently massage into the scalp. Take another few drops and massage into the rest of your hair down to the ends. Only a few drops are needed for most hair types, more for overly dry or coarse hair. Can be applied to wet or dry hair.

Yield: 3 ounces (60 ml)

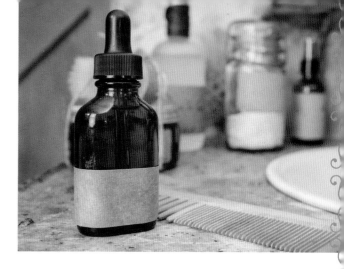

Conditioning Treatment Oil

This extremely moisturizing oil leaves the hair soft, shiny, and manageable. You can also customize this recipe by adding essential oils for any scalp ailment, oily or thinning hair, or dandruff by following the relevant directions below.

INGREDIENTS

¼ cup (60 ml) avocado oil
¼ cup (60 ml) olive oil
¼ cup (60 ml) broccoli seed oil
¼ cup (60 ml) watermelon seed oil
5 drops rosemary essential oil
5 drops chamomile essential oil
5 drops lavender essential oil

FOR OILY HAIR:

5 drops each of lemon balm essential oil, lemongrass essential oil, rosemary essential oil, and tea tree essential oil

FOR DANDRUFF:

5 drops each of basil essential oil, cedarwood essential oil, juniper essential oil, patchouli essential oil, tea tree essential oil, and thyme essential oil

FOR THINNING HAIR:

5 drops each of cedarwood essential oil, geranium essential oil, grapefruit essential oil, juniper essential oil, neroli essential oil, rosemary essential oil, and thyme essential oil

DIRECTIONS

Combine all the ingredients, mix well, and store in a sterile container. This recipe can be doubled and stored away from heat and direct sunlight for up to 3 months.

To use, while the hair is still damp, apply a small amount to your fingertips and gently massage into the scalp. Take another few drops and massage into the rest of your hair down to the ends. For best results, pin up your hair and leave the oil in for at least 20 minutes. Gentle heat can also be applied to enhance the results.

This can also be applied to the scalp as a massage treatment oil; simply apply a few drops to the fingertips and massage into the scalp to increase circulation and stimulate hair growth. They can even be left in overnight for added effectiveness

Yield: 1 cup (235 ml)

↣ HERBAL COLOR RINSES ↢

Herbal infusions can also help enhance natural hair color or refresh color-treated hair. Below are some herbs that can be used to create an infusion that can then be added to your regular shampoo to give your hair a color boost. If you don't have all the herbs available to you, it's okay to use any combination of the herbs. For example, blue malva flower on its own works great for blonde or gray hair to combat brassy hues.

Blonde hair	* * *	Blue malva, calendula, chamomile, lemon peel
Red hair	* * *	Calendula, cinnamon bark, hibiscus
Dark hair	* * *	Black tea, cinnamon, cloves, dried rosemary
Gray hair	* * *	Blue malva, rosemary, sage, thyme

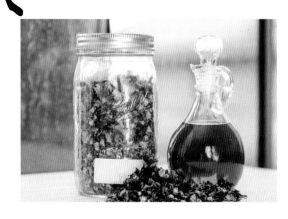

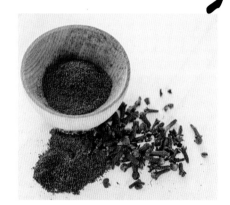

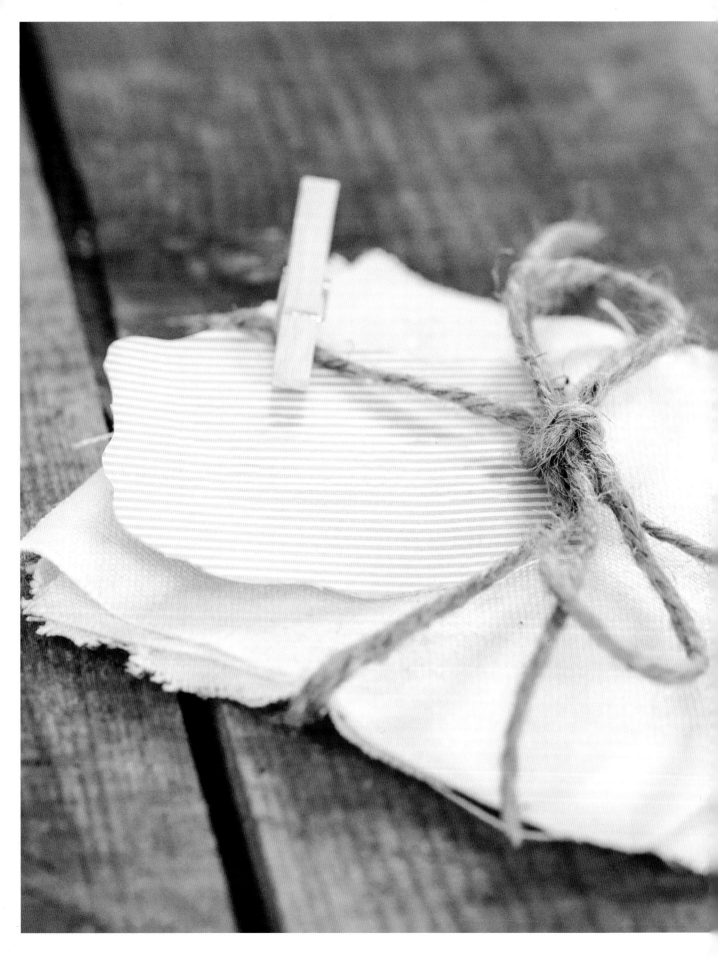

CHAPTER 7

Recipes for the Home

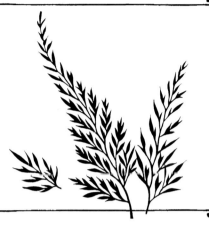

THE PRODUCTS WE USE IN OUR HOMES CAN BE JUST AS IMPORTANT TO OUR GENERAL WELL-BEING AS THE PRODUCTS WE USE IN AND ON OUR BODIES. THE USE OF TOXIC CLEANSERS AND PESTICIDES CAN GREATLY AFFECT OUR HEALTH AS WELL AS THE ENVIRONMENT. OUR HOME SHOULD BE A CONTINUAL SOURCE OF STRENGTH AND HEALING. THIS CHAPTER, THROUGH AROMATHERAPY AND GREEN ALTERNATIVES TO CLEANING, WILL HELP YOU CREATE A BALANCED, HEALTHY HOME.

→ KITCHEN RESCUES ←

Here are some quick home care rescues that you'll find in your kitchen:

* **Lemon:** Use it to clean and polish chrome.

* **Sliced grapefruit, lemons, and oranges:** Simmer in a pot of water for an hour or so; this will not only freshen the house but will also clean aluminum pots.

* **Vinegar:** Add it to your clothing wash to help remove dirt and odors.

Aromatherapy is the practice of using pure essential oils for their therapeutic, aromatic, healing properties. We humans are able to distinguish among more than 10,000 different odor molecules. Our sense of smell can trigger memories, attract us to our mates, select the foods we like or dislike, and affect our mood. Aroma causes a variety of chemical reactions in our bodies. Because of this, aromatherapy can be used to treat a multitude of ailments. There are many ways to expose yourself to aromatherapy; we've already discussed a lot of them in the earlier recipes for topical applications. Diffusing is another method for releasing the powers of essential oils into the air, and there are many ways to do this, including with a simple room spray or a diffusion ring or by adding them to a bowl of water.

Below is a list of essential oils for aromatherapy. For more in-depth essential oil information, please refer to chapter 2.

Calming and relaxing: Basil, bergamot, chamomile, geranium, jasmine, lavender, lemongrass, neroli, ravensara, rosewood, sandalwood, ylang ylang

Depression: Anise, bergamot, chamomile, cinnamon, clary sage, cypress, geranium, grapefruit, juniper, lavender, lemon, neroli, patchouli, peppermint, rosemary

Stress relieving: Angelica, basil, cedarwood, chamomile, cypress, geranium, jasmine, lavender, lemon, neroli, petitgrain, rose, ylang ylang

Uplifting: Clary sage, cypress, eucalyptus, grapefruit, juniper, lemon, lime, mandarin, peppermint, ylang ylang

Nausea: Basil, chamomile, dill, ginger, lavender, lemon, peppermint

Hangover: Cedarwood, grapefruit, juniper, lavender, lemon, rosemary

CLEANING SUPPLIES

With tons of commercial household cleansers on the market today we are often swayed by the promise of a sanitized, fresh-smelling home. What we don't realize is the chemicals used to do so are often hazardous, are corrosive to surfaces (especially our skin), and pollute the air. Nature once again can provide us with some clever, quick, and easy alternatives to harsh cleansers. The following recipes will clean and refresh your home without the harsh side effects of commercial products.

Kitchen Sink Scrub

No need for harsh chemical abrasives and bleach; baking soda and white vinegar can handle almost any stain you throw at them, while disinfecting at the same time.

INGREDIENTS

½ cup (112 g) baking soda
¼ cup (60 ml) white vinegar
5 drops lime essential oil
5 drops lemon essential oil

DIRECTIONS

In a bowl, mix all the ingredients together.

To use, spoon the mixture onto a sponge or washcloth and scrub the area to be cleaned.

Yield: ¾ cup (170 g)

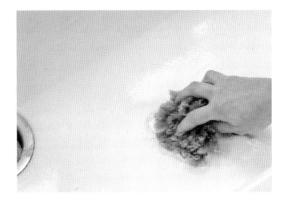

Household Disinfecting Cleanser

This is a great cleanser to use around flu season. Just bottle this mixture in a spray bottle and it can work as an all-purpose cleanser throughout the house.

INGREDIENTS

1 cup (235 ml) white vinegar
2 cups (470 ml) distilled water
20 drops lemon essential oil
20 drops eucalyptus essential oil
10 drops tea tree essential oil

DIRECTIONS

Combine all the ingredients in a spray bottle.

To use, spray onto surface to be cleaned and wipe dry using either paper towels or a sponge. For more effective cleaning, let sit on the surface for at least a minute or more before wiping dry.

Yield: 3 cups (705 ml)

Carpet Deodorizer

Great for homes with pets, this recipe freshens the carpet and home. It will also keep your vacuum smelling great.

INGREDIENTS

15 drops elemi essential oil

15 drops geranium essential oil

15 drops peppermint essential oil

3 cups (675 g) baking soda

DIRECTIONS

In a bowl, slowly add the essential oils to the baking soda and mix well. Once fully blended, pour into a shaker-top container, if available, or place in a sealable container and apply with a large slotted spoon.

To use, shake onto the carpet. Leave on the carpet for up to an hour before vacuuming.

Yield: 3 cups (675 g)

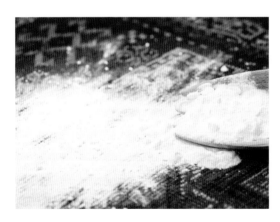

Mold and Mildew Treatment

Use this treatment in areas of your home or garden that are prone to mildew and mold buildup. It's great to use in the bathroom and on terra-cotta garden pots.

INGREDIENTS

2 cups (77 g) fresh thyme, or 1 cup (43 g) dried

2½ to 3½ cups (588 to 822 ml) water

10 drops patchouli essential oil

10 drops cinnamon essential oil

10 drops tea tree essential oil

10 drops niaouli essential oil

DIRECTIONS

Make an herbal infusion with the thyme and water (see page 53). Let cool slightly, then add the essential oils. Transfer to a sealable container.

To use, wet a sponge or rag with the solution and wash down problem areas; let dry.

Yield: 2½ to 3½ cups (588 to 822 ml)

HOUSEHOLD INSECT DETERRENTS

Commercial pesticides can be extremely harmful to both our bodies and the environment. Essentials oils can provide effective yet healthy alternatives to store-bought bug repellents, plus they smell a lot better.

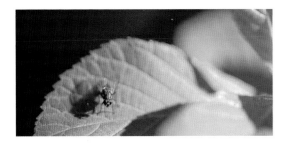

Fly Deterrent

Keep the flies at bay with this extremely simple recipe.

INGREDIENTS

1 cup (235 ml) water
30 drops peppermint essential oil

DIRECTIONS

Mix the ingredients together in a spray bottle.

To use, spray near doors, windows, countertops, and other areas where flies may be an issue.

Yield: 1 cup (235 ml)

Drawer Refresher and Moth Deterrent

This recipe does double duty as a natural drawer refresher while keeping the moths away.

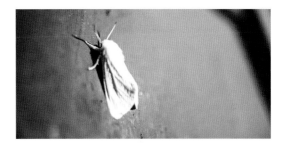

INGREDIENTS

1½ cups (355 ml) water
10 drops spearmint essential oil
10 drops lavender essential oil
10 drops lemongrass essential oil
10 drops cedarwood essential oil
10 drops clove essential oil
10 drops rosemary essential oil

DIRECTIONS

Mix the ingredients together in a sealable container. Take linen or muslin fabric (any absorbent fabric can be used, even old dishtowels or cloth napkins) and cut into small squares, about the size of a standard dryer sheet.

Dip the cloths into the mixture and hang up to dry on a clothing line or pin to a shower curtain.

Once the squares have dried they are ready to use.

To use, place in drawers or closets to keep away moths. Refresh the cloths as needed with more of the solution.

Yield: 1½ cups (355 ml)

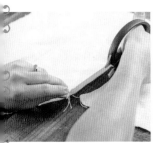
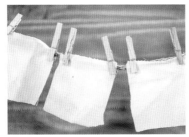
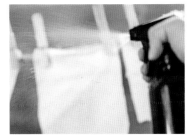
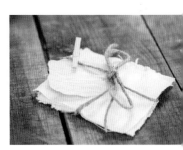

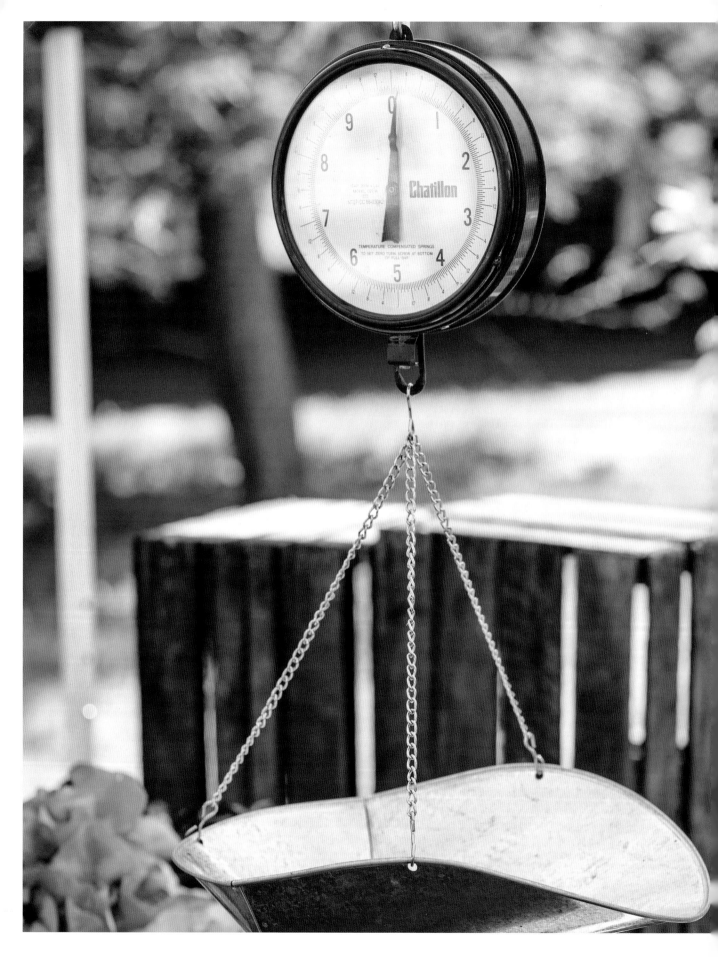

CHAPTER 8

Seasonal Recipes Inspired by Your Farmers' Market

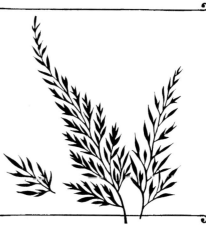

FARMERS' MARKETS CAN BE A GREAT SOURCE FOR AN APOTHECARY'S INSPIRATIONS. WHILE WE KNOW THAT FRUITS AND VEGETABLES ARE GOOD FOR US NUTRITIONALLY, WE SHOULDN'T FORGET THAT THEY CAN ALSO BE NOURISHING TO OUR OUTER BODIES. THIS CHAPTER'S RECIPES ARE SEPARATED BY SEASON, BUT BE CREATIVE WITH WHAT'S AVAILABLE.

In chapter 4 you'll find some recipes for powdered cleansers. As discussed, powdered cleansers can be mixed with a variety of wetting agents, such as water and fruit juice. Following are some great food-inspired wetting agents that, depending on the season, you can pick up at your local farmers' market. Get inspired by what is in season—don't limit your creativity!

Sensitive Skin	Dry Skin	Normal Skin	Oily or Acne-prone Skin
Apple juice with a chamomile and rose petal infusion	Cantaloupe juice with lemon balm infusion	Raspberry juice with raspberry leaf infusion	Tomato juice with garlic infusion

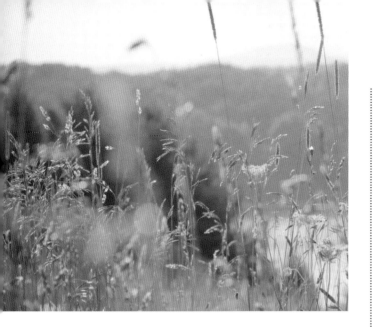

SUMMER

Summer is the time we most often think of going to our local farmers' market, when, depending on your location, vegetable and herbs are most abundant. When shopping for the ingredients for tonight's dinner, don't forget that there are many fruits, vegetables, and herbs that can be made into beautifying skin care recipes.

Carrot Age-Defying Mask

Rich in antioxidant beta-carotene, this mask nourishes the skin, giving it a radiant glow.

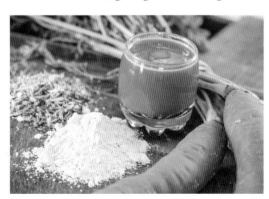

INGREDIENTS

⅓ cup (80 ml) fresh organic carrot juice
2 tablespoons (16 g) kaolin clay
2 tablespoons (16 g) green tea leaf powder

DIRECTIONS

Combine all the ingredients in a small bowl to create a paste.

To use, apply the paste to the face and neck, avoiding the eye area. Leave the mask on the skin for 10 to 15 minutes, and then rinse with warm water.

Yield: 1 mask

Basil and Lemon Balm Relaxing Herbal Infusion

Whether you grab these herbs from your summer garden or from the local farmers' market, this herbal tonic will settle an upset stomach or reduce anxiety and stress.

INGREDIENTS

1 part fresh basil
1 part fresh lemon balm
Honey, to taste (optional)

DIRECTIONS

Make an herbal infusion with the basil and lemon balm (see page 53). Add honey, if desired.

To use, drink 3 to 4 cups (705 to 940 ml) daily until the conditions subsides.

Cucumber Toner

This toner is great for soothing and tightening the skin, diminishing puffiness.

INGREDIENTS

1 or 2 organic cucumbers, peeled and chopped
¼ cup (60 ml) witch hazel
¼ cup (60 ml) distilled water

DIRECTIONS

Place all the ingredients in a blender and purée until smooth and well blended. Strain the mixture using a fine-mesh strainer. Use a spatula or the back of a spoon to push the liquid out, and pour it into a sterile container. This blend should be stored in the refrigerator.

To use, apply to the face using a cotton ball and then follow with moisturizer. Or for a refreshing summer mist, store in a spray bottle and spray the face throughout the day whenever the skin needs a little pick-me-up.

Yield: 1 cup (235 ml)

Pineapple Papaya Body Exfoliator

Not only does it taste good, but pineapple is also extremely beneficial to both the inside and the outside of your body. Containing the enzyme bromelain, a natural exfoliant, pineapple makes an amazing body scrub. Papaya, rich in skin-hydrating antioxidants, contains papain, which is helpful for removing dead skin cells.

INGREDIENTS

¼ cup (40 g) diced pineapple
¼ cup (44 g) diced papaya
1 tablespoon (15 ml) jojoba oil (optional, for added moisture)
2 tablespoons (25 g) coarse sugar or coarse Dead Sea salt

DIRECTIONS

In a blender, purée the pineapple, papaya, and jojoba oil until completely blended and smooth. Stir in the sugar and pour into a sterile container. Store in the refrigerator.

To use, while in the shower, using either your fingertips or a loofah sponge, gently massage the scrub onto the skin, then rinse. Pat dry.

Yield: ½ cup (85 g)

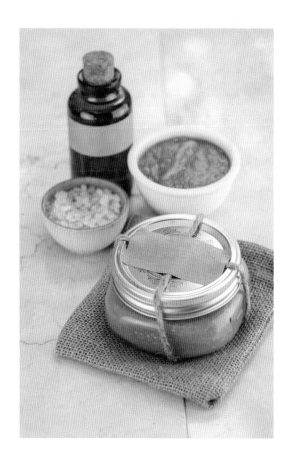

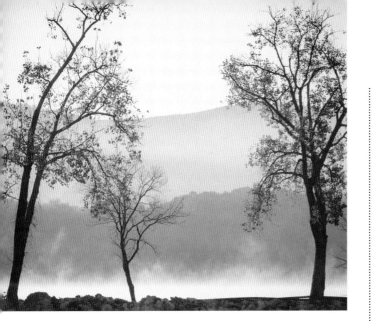

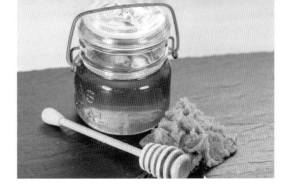

Autumn

Has the air started to get colder? All the aromas and flavors we crave in the fall can also be used as scrubs, masks, and more.

Skin-Smoothing Apple Body Scrub

This scrub not only smells amazing enough to eat, but it's great for the skin, too. The apples and apricot act as a gentle moisturizer while the antimicrobial abilities of honey and clove cleanse the skin. The brown sugar gently scrubs away dead skin cells and impurities.

INGREDIENTS

```
6 apples of your choice, or what's
  available at your farmers' market,
  peeled, cored, and chopped
1/2 cup (120 ml) apricot kernel oil
1/4 cup (80 g) honey
1 tablespoon (8 g) clove powder, or
  10 drops clove essential oil
1 tablespoon (15 ml) freshly squeezed
  orange juice
1 cup (225 g) coarse brown sugar
```

DIRECTIONS

In a blender, purée the apples. You may need to add some of the oil to get the mixture moving in the blender. Transfer to a mixing bowl, add the remaining ingredients, and stir to combine. Transfer to a sterile sealable container. Store in the refrigerator.

To use, while in the shower, using either your fingertips or a loofah sponge, gently massage the scrub onto the skin, then rinse. Pat dry.

Yield: 2 cups (470 ml)

Pumpkin Mask

This simple yet effective mask hydrates and tightens the skin.

INGREDIENTS

```
1 small pumpkin
1/4 cup (80 g) honey
```

DIRECTIONS

Remove the skin and seeds from the pumpkin. Chop it and boil or roast to soften. Let cool. Transfer to a blender or food processor and purée, then add the honey and mix again. Transfer to a sterile sealable container. Store in the refrigerator.

To use, apply the cool mixture to the face, leave on for at least 20 minutes, then rinse and pat dry.

Yield: 3 or 4 applications

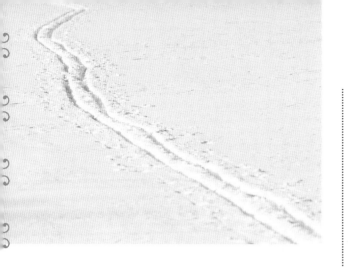

WINTER

Winter is usually the time that it becomes harder to source local ingredients and also when our skin is most in need of pampering. If you can't get to a farmers' market, look for local produce at your grocery store.

Oily Skin Orange Facial Mask

Orange is a great source of vitamin C, an excellent antiaging vitamin, and enhances collagen production while removing excess oil and preventing inflammation. Honey, a natural humectant, is a fantastic antiseptic and is great for cleansing the skin.

INGREDIENTS
Juice from 1 fresh orange
½ cup (60 g) arrowroot powder
1 teaspoon honey

DIRECTIONS
Combine all the ingredients in a bowl to create a paste.

To use, apply to the face and leave on for 20 minutes. Rinse with warm water and pat dry.

Yield: 1 mask

Potato Cleanser

Potatoes are thought to have many medicinal properties. This cleanser absorbs oils and leaves the skin clean and refreshed.

INGREDIENTS
¼ cup (28 g) chopped potato (skin on)
¼ cup (60 g) yogurt
1 egg
½ teaspoon baking soda

DIRECTIONS
In a blender, purée the potato. You may need to add some yogurt or the egg to get the machine moving. Add the remaining ingredients one at a time until blended. Store in the refrigerator.

To use, apply the cleanser with your fingertips in a circular motion. Rinse with warm water and follow with toner and moisturizer.

Yield: 1 or 2 applications

Potato Slices Dark Circle and Puffiness Treatment

Here's another great use for potatoes, which, when sliced, help alleviate dark or puffy circles under your eyes.

INGREDIENTS
2 potato slices

DIRECTIONS
Place the potato slices over the eyes while lying down, and leave on for 20 to 30 minutes.

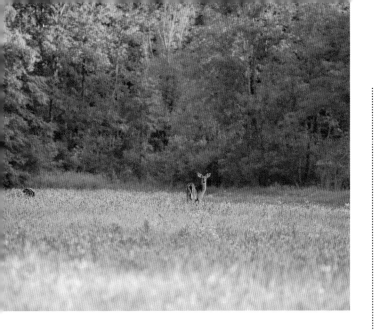

Spring

This is the time we start to come out of hibernation; this goes for fruits, vegetables, and herbs, too. Farmers' markets start to become easier to find and have much more inventory. Spring is also the time when we often start taking care of bodies again, with renewed exercise routines and attention to nutrition. Our skin is often in need of a reboot, too, from the drying, dulling effects of winter.

Skin Lightening and Brightening Shiitake Mushroom Toner

Rich in kojic acid, mushrooms have become popular not only for healthy eating but also for skin care. Kojic acid brightens skin tone and fades freckles, scars, and sun damage.

INGREDIENTS

6 shiitake mushrooms
3 cups (705 ml) water
1 teaspoon vegetable glycerin
4 drops lavender essential oil
2 drops chamomile essential oil

DIRECTIONS

Bring the mushrooms and water to a boil in a saucepan and let simmer for 20 to 30 minutes. Strain the liquid into a sterile container and let cool. Add the glycerin and essential oils and shake to combine. Store in the refrigerator.

To use, apply to the solution to a cotton ball and gently wipe the face. Follow with a moisturizer.

Yield: 2 cups (470 ml)

Avocado Hair Mask

Hydrating to both the scalp and the hair, this nourishing mask repairs, strengthens, and adds shine and softness.

INGREDIENTS

1 ripe avocado
¼ cup (60 ml) jojoba oil

DIRECTIONS

Cut open the avocado, remove the pit, scoop the flesh into a bowl, and mash with a fork. Add the jojoba oil and mix well.

To use, apply the mask to damp hair and scalp, pin your hair up, and put on a shower cap. After 20 minutes, rinse off the mask and follow with a gentle shampoo. Dry and style as usual.

Yield: 1 mask

Plum Face Mask

Rich in antioxidants, this mask works to protect the skin from damaging UV rays and hydrates while also absorbing oils.

INGREDIENTS

6 plums
1 tablespoon (15 ml) jojoba oil

DIRECTIONS

Add the plums to a pan of water, bring to a boil over high heat, and cook until soft. Strain the plums from the water, transfer to a bowl, and let cool. Once cool, remove the skins and pits and place the flesh in a blender. Add the jojoba oil and purée well.

To use, apply the mask with your fingertips in a gentle circular motion; leave on for 15 to 20 minutes, then rinse and pat dry. Follow with a toner and moisturizer.

Yield: 1 mask

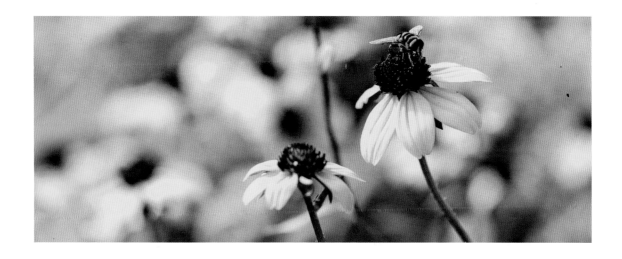

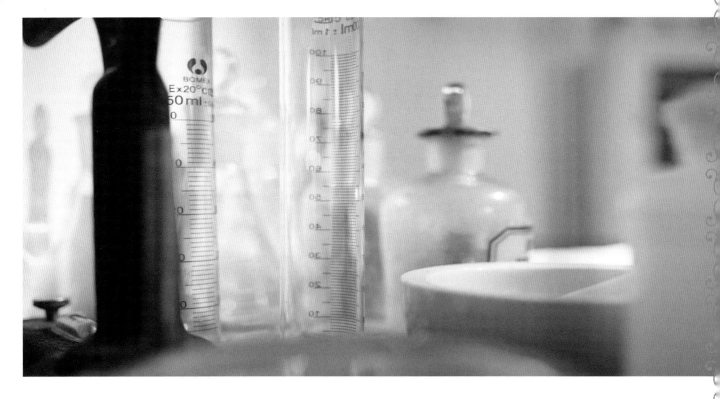

Appendix

Quick Reference Charts

Following are quick reference charts that may come in handy when you are making and using the recipes in this book or creating your own.

→ SUBSTITUTIONS FOR COMMON INGREDIENTS ←

These are some substitutes for ingredients in case you don't have them on hand.

Ingredient		Substitute
Borax		Baking soda
Glycerin		Honey
Lanolin		Coconut oil
Arrowroot or rice flour		Cornstarch
Stearic acid		Beeswax
Vodka		Witch hazel

→ DOSAGE GUIDELINES ←

Here are some basic dosage guidelines for both the recipes in this book and those that you make up. Please keep in mind that they are only guidelines and can vary according to the recipe and plant material used.

Recipe Type	Suggested Dilution (this may vary depending on the recipe and oil used)
Massage oil	10 to 30 drops per 1 ounce (30 ml) carrier oil
Compress	3 to 5 drops per ¼ cup (60 ml) water
Bath soak	5 to 10 drops in bathwater
Room diffuser (aromatherapy)	3 to 5 drops per small bowl of water
Face oil (lotion) / Body oil (lotion)	5 to 10 drops / 10 to 20 drops per 1 ounce (30 ml) of carrier oil

Remedy Type	Standard Adult Dosages
Infusions and teas	1 cup (235 ml) 3 times daily
Decoctions	1 cup (235 ml) 3 times daily
Syrups	¼ teaspoon every 4 hours until symptoms subside
Tinctures	½ teaspoon 3 times daily
Compresses	10 to 15 minutes at a time as needed (for no longer than 2 days)
Poultices	2 or 3 times a day for 2 hours at a time (for no longer than 2 days)
Steam inhalations	2 or 3 times a day for up to 10 minutes at a time

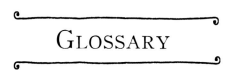

GLOSSARY

Alchemy (alchemist): early form of chemistry that sought to change base metals into gold, discover cures, and create potions to cure all diseases.

Allergen: any substance that can cause an allergic reaction.

Analgesic: a substance capable of reducing or eliminating pain.

Antibacterial: the ability to inhibit the growth of bacteria.

Antifungal: the ability to inhibit the growth of fungi.

Anti-inflammatory: the ability to reduce swelling.

Antimicrobial: the ability to inhibit the growth of microbes.

Antioxidant: a substance, vitamin, or mineral that inhibits the effects of aging of the skin by free radicals.

Antiseptic: the ability to clean or be free of germs.

Aromatherapy: the use of scent or fragrance to affect mood, behavior, and health.

Astringent: a substance that cleans the skin and minimizes pore size.

Botany: the study of plant life.

Bronchial: consisting of the throat and bronchial tubes.

Carcinogen: a substance believed to cause cancer.

Carrier oil: an oil, derived from either a plant or a nut, used to dilute essential oils and that is absolutely for safe application and skin penetration.

Collagen: a protein found in the body that connects and supports skin, bones, tendons, and cartilage.

Compress: a cloth used to apply pressure, heat, cold, a poultice, or a medication to an area, usually for an extended period of time.

Decoction: the extraction of substances (plant material) by boiling.

Dermatitis: inflammation of the skin.

Detoxification: the removal of harmful toxins.

Diuretic: a substance or an agent that increases the flow of fluids.

Eczema: a condition of the skin that causes extremely dry skin, lesions, redness, itching, and burning.

Effleurage: a form of extraction by movement or massage.

Emulsifier: a substance that holds together or prevents the separation of two immiscible liquids.

Emulsion: the combination of two immiscible liquids (oil and water) into one.

Endocrine disruptor: a chemical that mimics or interferes with the body's hormones and can cause reproductive or neurological damage.

Exfoliate: to remove dead skin scales from the face or body.

Herbal infusion: to steep plant material in hot water to extract its medicinal properties.

Humectant: a substance that has the ability to produce or retain moisture.

Impurities: contaminants, toxins, or pollutants.

Maceration: to soften or separate by soaking.

Medicinal: to have therapeutic or healing properties.

Ointment: an oily, emollient substance applied to the skin for medicinal or cosmetic purposes. Also known as a salve or balm.

Phytochemicals: plant-based material believed to have beneficial medicinal and cosmetic effects.

Poultice: a soft, usually heated, herbal medicinal blend spread on cloth and applied to skin to aid the healing of sores, lesions, and inflammation.

Preservative: a substance that preserves, fighting bacteria, decomposition, or fermentation in another substance.

Salve: an oily, emollient substance applied to the skin for medicinal or cosmetic purposes. Also known as an ointment or a balm.

Solvent: a substance that is capable of dissolving another substance.

Solvent extraction: the extraction of one liquid into another liquid.

Steam distillation: the separation process for temperature-sensitive materials.

Sulfate: a salt or an ester of sulfuric acid; in shampoo it is most often the detergent or lathering agent.

Tincture: a concentrated liquid extract of plant material using alcohol, vinegar, or vegetable glycerin as the solvent.

Tonic: a medicinal blend intended to improve, invigorate, and strengthen the body and improve overall health.

RESOURCES

★ WEBSITES ★

THE CAMPAIGN FOR SAFE COSMETICS
www.safecosmetics.org
A great resource regarding harmful chemicals in cosmetics and personal care products and safer alternatives.

ENVIRONMENTAL WORKING GROUP'S SKIN DEEP DATABASE
www.ewg.org/skindeep
An amazing resource for ingredient information. Any time I use a new product or consider a new ingredient for a recipe, I always double-check it here.

MAKE YOUR COSMETICS.COM
www.makeyourcosmetics.com
Recipes and information for at-home cosmetics.

ORGANIC BEAUTY CARE RECIPES
www.organic-beauty-recipes.com
DIY recipes for face, hair, and body.

★ INGREDIENT SUPPLIERS ★

100% P.E.O
www.100pureessentialoils.com
A great resource for 100 percent pure essential oils and supplies.

THE ESSENTIAL OIL COMPANY
www.essentialoil.com
Essential oils, distillation equipment, and soaps.

FROM NATURE WITH LOVE
www.fromnaturewithlove.com
One of my favorite ingredients suppliers. They are also a great information and recipe resource.

FRONTIER NATURAL PRODUCTS CO-OP
www.frontiercoop.com
Herbs, essential oils, supplies, and more.

JEAN'S GREENS
www.jeansgreens.com
Essential oils, extract elixirs, and herbs.

STARWEST BOTANICALS
www.starwest-botanicals.com
Bulk herbs, oils, teas, and natural products.

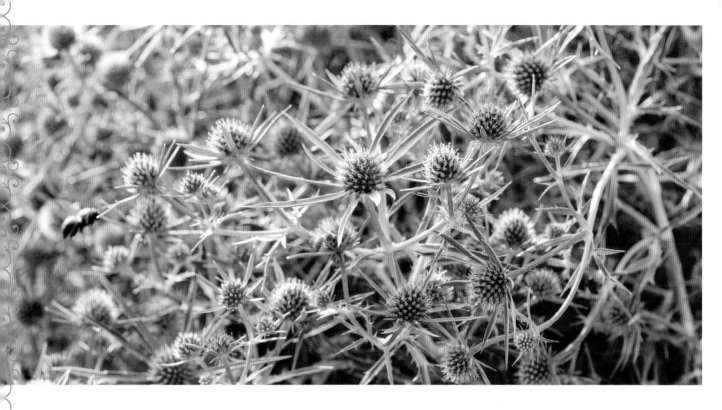

ACKNOWLEDGMENTS

First and foremost, I'd like to thank my amazing husband for his continued support and encouragement. Without his belief in my ideas and dreams, along with his willingness to always be my product guinea pig, I could have never accomplished what I have today. You are my rock. Thank you.

Jacsen, you were with me for every moment of this book, and I thank you for being the perfect son.

To my family, Jennifer and Fergal, whose generosity and encouragement help make it all possible. Mom, thank you for your support in all my endeavors throughout the years. Elaine, thank you for your time and beautiful face.

To my editor Tiffany, thank you so much for your direction, support, insight, and extreme patience in making this book. You were such a delight to work with.

To Natalie and Kira, without your hard work, patience, and loyalty throughout the writing of this book, I would have had to close the shop doors! You're truly the best, and I'm grateful every day for you both.

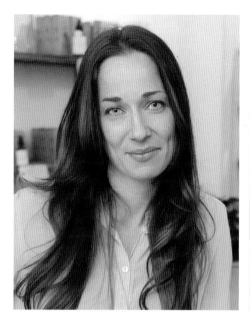
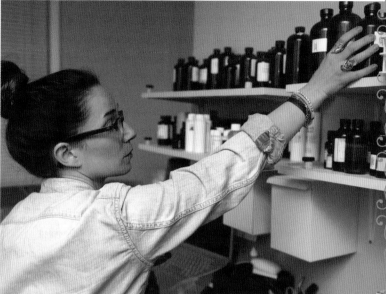

ABOUT THE AUTHOR

Stacey Dugliss-Wesselman, founder of Cold Spring Apothecary, started crafting her remedies as a child growing up in the Catskill Mountains. Her interests in biology, chemistry, and naturals continued into adulthood, and she pursued a career in nursing and later cosmetology. Working in Brooklyn, New York, as a stylist, she began mixing her concoctions for her clients. After much encouragement from family and friends, Stacey created the line of products from which Cold Spring Apothecary was born. Driven by an allergy from the harsh parabens and drying sulfates found in modern-day cosmetics, Stacey first created her shampoos, which are now best sellers. Her passion for naturals led her to create a full line of hair care products, from cleansing shampoos to styling aids and scalp treatments.

To date, the line of products has grown to include treatments for the skin, hair, body, and home. Stacey has a strong belief in educating the consumer. Cold Spring Apothecary products are crafted by hand and have an innate sense of luxury that keeps her customers wanting more.

Cold Spring Apothecary products became available for purchase online in 2010. The first flagship location opened in April 2011 in the historic village of its namesake. Her products have garnered a cult-like following with mass appeal and can now be found across the United States and Canada in select boutiques and salons.

INDEX

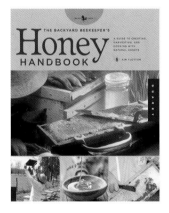

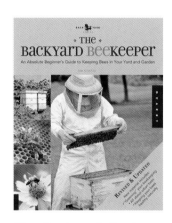

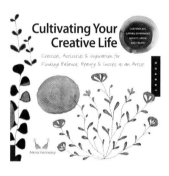

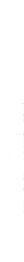